CIRCUMCISION

CIRCUMCISION

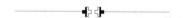

A HISTORY OF THE

WORLD'S MOST

CONTROVERSIAL SURGERY

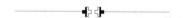

DAVID L. GOLLAHER

BASIC BOOKS

A MEMBER OF THE PERSEUS BOOKS GROUP

Published by Basic Books,
A Member of the Perseus Books Group

Library of Congress Cataloging-in-Publication Data

Gollaher, David, 1949–
Circumcision: a history of the world's most controversial surgery / David L. Gollaher.
p.   cm.
Includes index.
ISBN 0-465-04397-6
1. Circumcision—History.   I. Title.

GT2470.G65 2000
392.21—dc21

Book design by Victoria Kuskowski

FOR MY PARENTS

CONTENTS

ACKNOWLEDGMENTS

Circumcision, persisting for thousands of years, flowing from tribal rituals through the world's great religions into modern medicine, presents the historian with an unusual array of challenges. In trying to manage them, I've incurred a variety of fortunate debts.

First, I had a chance to develop and present in a preliminary way the idea that medical circumcision in the United States was a product of profound social and cultural forces. I published "From Ritual to Science: The Medical Transformation of Circumcision in America" in the *Journal of Social History*, and I benefited greatly from editor Peter N. Stearns's comments and questions. Subsequently, over the course of the next few years, I engaged in extended, wide-ranging discussions with historians Ronald L. Numbers, Donald Fleming, William R. Hutchison, Howard Kushner, Andrew Scull, and with John Seely Brown, the polymath director of Xerox Palo Alto Research Center.

As I became more intrigued with the continuing controversy surrounding neonatal circumcision, and began to wade through the immense body of medical research on the subject, I enjoyed help from a distinguished group of physicians and surgeons. These include my former colleagues at Scripps Clinic, Roger Cornell, Ruben Gittes, Peter Walther, and the late Tony Moore. George W. Kaplan, a pediatric urologist who served on the American Academy of Pediatrics Task Force on Circumcision, was generous with his time and suggestions, helping balance my account.

Activists opposing what they consider genital mutilation are integral to the story told here. Among them, Marilyn Milos and Tim Hammond were especially helpful in explaining their cause and providing source materials.

Of the many libraries and archives I visited in search of evidence, I recall with special gratitude the staffs at Harvard Medical School's Countway Library, the National Library of Medicine, the Biomedical Library at the University of California, San Diego, and the Centro Internazionale per la Storia delle Universitá e della Scienza at the Universitá di Bologna.

Editor William Frucht at Basic Books played a critical role both in helping refine my argument and in clarifying my prose. My literary agents Glen Hartley and Lynn Chu contributed not just their commercial expertise but good ideas and encouragement at every stage.

Any attempt to describe the contributions of my wife Moya Gollaher would be partial and inadequate. Suffice it to say that she inspires the world of her husband and children with energy, intellectual curiosity, humor, and common sense. These are qualities that improve an author's life and, I hope, have found their way into this book.

D.G.
La Jolla, California
September 1999

PREFACE

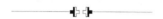

Circumcision is the oldest enigma in the history of surgery. It is far easier to imagine the impulse behind Neolithic cave painting than to guess what inspired the ancients to cut their genitals or the genitals of their young. Yet millennia ago, long before medicine and religion branched into separate streams of wisdom — indeed, long before history itself — cutting the foreskin of the penis was invented as a symbolic wound; thus circumcision became a ritual of extraordinary power.

Some groups adopted circumcision as a divine injunction, a mark of the gods, or of God. To outsiders the practice seemed inexplicable. Why, Greeks wondered derisively of Jews, would any people routinely mutilate their young? In time the mystery lessened, though not because the surgery disappeared. It merely became familiar, an essential feature of Judaism and Islam, and then in modern times, of Anglo-American medicine.

Still, familiarity scarcely resolved the riddle of circumcision. Down through the ages, the operation's ritual and religious meanings remained cloaked in obscurity. As for medical circumcision, which swept America and Britain around the turn of the twentieth century, physicians and laypeople alike remain ferociously divided about the risks, benefits, and ethics of the procedure. Mountains of research have produced no general agreement about the medical evidence. Indeed, the ongoing battle between advocates and opponents of circumcision bears out William Osler's dictum that in such disputes, "the greater the ignorance, the greater the dogmatism."

This book is a history, not a polemic nor a tract for the times. Throughout, I've endeavored to write a balanced account that accurately reflects what people, at different times, thought and did. The historian Carl Becker once described history quite elegantly as providing "the artificial extension of social memory." In this instance, I'm interested in reaching deep into the past, to the very limits of social memory, and, at the same time, exploring the history of the present to chronicle the patterns of thought and behavior that characterize circumcision in the present age.

Historians typically strive to make the strange familiar. But I hope also to make the familiar strange. What people take for granted is not necessarily natural. In the United States, circumcision of newborns is so common that most parents and physicians scarcely think of it as surgery. Yet for most of the twentieth century it has remained the most frequently performed surgical procedure in America. For the majority of newborn American males, a surgeon cuts off the foreskin with little more thought than severing the umbilical cord. As a medical norm, this contrasts sharply with most other industrialized nations, where physicians seldom perform the operation except to treat manifest disorders.

But attitudes in the United States are changing. One reason is that a vocal and growing minority of pediatricians and family physicians now openly dispute the wisdom of operating on the genitals of healthy infants. Readers of leading medical journals realize that there is no conclusive scientific evidence in favor of a routine operation. After scouring the medical literature, the American Academy of Pediatrics' Task Force on Circumcision reported in 1999, "Existing scientific evidence supports potential benefits of newborn circumcision; however these data are not sufficient to recommend routine neonatal circumcision." In the wake of this statement, a chorus of critics pointed out that, even if circumcision offered some slight statistical advantages, surgery in the absence of disease violated Hippocrates' sacred dictum: *primum non nocere.** Even so, advocates for circumcision remained unconvinced, likening the operation to a kind of vaccination that offered a lifetime of protection against cancer, urinary tract infections, sexually transmitted diseases, and even AIDS.

Despite the enduring controversy, proponents seem to be fighting a losing battle. Skeptics include most modern medical communities outside the United States, and many American baby-boom parents, well educated, steeped in 1960s suspicion of professional authority, who are voicing qualms of their own. Their questions represent a fusion of physical, psychological, and cultural concerns. Is circumcision necessary for good hygiene? Does it help prevent diseases? What are the risks of complications from the operation itself? How about the pain? And, perhaps more important than anything else, do uncircumcised boys risk being stigmatized in the locker room because they look different from their schoolmates, or, for that matter, from their fathers?

With respect to medical practice, circumcision recalls a profound challenge that has haunted medicine since its beginnings. How can we know what

---

*"First, do no harm."

works best and what doesn't? How firmly rooted in science is what we do in the clinic? In what precisely does sufficient proof of effectiveness consist? The recent history of circumcision forces us to confront an uncomfortable truth, well captured by David Eddy, a leading expert on medical evidence. "It's really quite amazing, but after hundreds of years, in fact, I would estimate that only about ten to twenty percent of medical practices have been evaluated properly. What that means for the patient — and not just the patient but for the physician — is that for a large proportion of practices we really don't know what the outcomes or what the effects are."[1]

The intellectual problem in medicine is that, like many other procedures, the practice of circumcision is based not in science but in something else: tradition, experience, ritual.

One of the fascinating problems in the history of anthropology is how disconnected people in different parts of the world assigned meaning to genital cutting. Yet this is a question to be asked not only of the central Australian tribesmen, carefully placing amputated foreskins in the totem-trees where human souls languish between their departure from a dying man and their rebirth in a child; it is to be asked as well of modern surgeons, operating on the infants' genitals in hopes of preventing diseases, and of a sociey that, trusting physicians to know best, follows their dictates.

Over its long history, circumcision has borne a variety of important meanings — distinguishing a priestly class, initiating boys into the community of men, signifying God's chosen people and, in an age captivated by the idea of scientific medicine, marking the circumcised as superior in health. Still, while there are many understandable religious, cultural and aesthetic reasons men or parents might choose circumcision, it lacks a persuasive medical basis. Far from a hard science, medical practice is like a reef, with new practices growing, experimentally, every day, older practices getting choked out, and others hardening into custom even though they're dead. Doctors who circumcise have faith in the operation because it rarely harms patients and is consistent with the way they see the world. But doctors have no way of knowing how much worse or better off, an individual child would have been without the surgery. Even assigning a statistical likelihood of future disease to a circumcised or uncircumcised baby depends largely on which studies you choose to believe.

As a simple test, I propose the following thought experiment. Imagine, for a moment, that circumcision had never caught on in America as a neonatal routine. In other words, suppose the United States were, say, like Norway. Next, imagine that a physician were to urge, in a talk at the annual meeting of the American Academy of Pediatrics, doctors to begin operating on the genitals of all baby boys shortly after birth in order to achieve marginally lower incidence of urinary tract infections and perhaps some other diseases. Of course no physician would dream of proposing such a thing today. The threshold for demonstrated effectiveness in surgery, particularly surgery on infants, is far too high.

Indeed, as the history of female circumcision suggests, if male circumcision were confined to developing nations, it would by now have emerged as an international *cause célèbre,* stirring passionate opposition from feminists, physicians, politicians, and the global human rights community. If routine medical circumcision didn't exist today, no one would dare to invent it. Yet it does exist. And owing to a long and curious history, it is so deeply embedded in certain cultures and worldviews that it is hard to recognize for what it is.

CIRCUMCISION

ONE

The Jewish Tradition

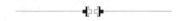

Every male among you shall be circumcised. You shall be circumcised in the flesh of your foreskins, and it shall be a sign of the covenant between me and you.

—*Genesis 17:10–11*

THE GENESIS OF CIRCUMCISION, LIKE MAGIC AND RELIGION, IS IMMEMORIAL. Evidence of its antiquity trails off in two distant streams. One of these flows from tribal societies, most famously, certain groups of Australian Aborigines, who have practiced totemic genital surgery for uncounted millennia. The other stream, far richer in historical materials yet equally mysterious with respect to its source, is a tributary into the mainstream of Western culture from the recesses of ancient Egypt.

The world's oldest account of circumcision is an image in an Egyptian tomb. On the West Bank of the Nile, across from Memphis, home of the legendary genius, architect and physician Imhotep, stands the necropolis of Saqqara. Even by Egyptian standards Saqqara is archaic, built sometime around 2400 B.C. during the Old Kingdom's fifth dynasty. There, inscribed on the walls of the royal tomb of Ankhmahor, one encounters a mélange of deities with ibis and beetle heads, humans, lions, cobras, and magical objects. Amidst these familiar representations, however, there is on the doorpost an extraordinary image: a well-preserved bas-relief of temple priests in the act of cutting the genitals of two young noblemen.

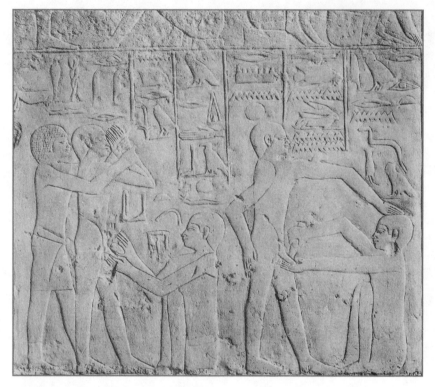

This bas-relief from the Egyptian necropolis at Saqqara (ca. 2400 B.C.) is the world's
most ancient depiction of a surgical operation. *Wellcome Institute Library.*

In the carving, the youths and priests are stylized figures. The tableaus strike
the modern eye as imaginary; but the bloody ordeal they represent was real
enough. In the first scene, an assistant stands behind one of the youths, gripping
his arms and pulling them back while the priest operates with a stone knife.
"Hold him and do not allow him to faint" reads the inscription. In the second
scene, the boy being circumcised urges the priest-surgeon to "thoroughly rub
off what is there." The circumcising priest replies, "I will cause it to heal." Performed on a child or adolescent, circumcision is exceptionally painful surgery—
twentieth-century doctors, when operating after infancy, ordinarily administer
a general anesthetic. The Egyptian ritual must have presented an opportunity for
a youth, on the threshold of manhood, to demonstrate his mastery over bodily
pain. Describing a mass circumcision ritual in the twenty-third century B.C., an
Egyptian named Uha boasted that he and his peers faced the ordeal with stoic
calm. "When I was circumcised, together with one hundred and twenty men,"
he recalled, "there was none thereof who hit out, there was none thereof who

was hit, and there was none thereof who scratched and there was none thereof who was scratched." That Uha remarked on the lack of hitting and scratching suggests, of course, that other ceremonies met with considerable resistance.[1]

The stele upon which Uha wrote his account and the wall carving in Ankhmahor are the earliest known records of circumcision. The historical trail begins with them. Yet what the Saqqara figures document was not the inception of a new ritual but a tradition far older than history itself. Mummified remains exhumed elsewhere in Egypt, predating Saqqara, have been subjected to X-ray scans, computerized tomography, and carbon dating. Some of these ancient corpses reveal indications of circumcision performed perhaps as early as 4000 B.C.[2]

The antiquity of circumcision, together with the fact that its social and religious significance in Egypt under the pharaohs has resisted convincing explanation, magnifies the mystery surrounding its origins. Beginning in the third millennium B.C., Egypt created a powerful mystique based in large measure on intellectual vitality and technological splendor. The Egyptians' advanced understanding of the human body, like their architectural prowess and military conquests, dazzled contemporaries and later generations alike. Whatever its symbolic meaning, the simple fact that Egyptians practiced circumcision invested the procedure with exceptional prestige in the ancient world. If the Egyptians excised the foreskin, many people reasoned, their motives must have been rooted in wisdom.

But what was that wisdom? Throughout history, religion has been humankind's instrument for ordering the world—and it centers on the idea of hierarchy. Religious ritual, in ways obvious and subtle, tend to reinforce an awareness of rank. Within the magico-religious framework of Egyptian science and medicine, circumcision apparently was a ritual marking the passage from youth to manhood. The transition was profound. Beyond the physical alteration of anatomy, the ritual entailed admittance into divine mysteries—secrets revealed only to the initiated. The content of these mysteries remains elusive, though they must have involved myths, prayers, and incantations central to Egyptian religion. The Egyptian Book of the Dead, for example, tells of the sun god Ra performing a self-circumcision, whose blood created two minor guardian deities.[3]

Egyptian thought drew no distinction between religion and medicine. Imhotep was revered as a physician and godlike healer. He was also the high priest at Heliopolis, an astrologer and wisdom figure whose reputation still inspired cult worship two millennia after his death.

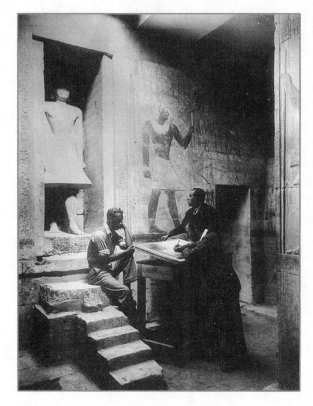

Members of the Saqqara
Expedition of the
Oriental Institute of the
University of Chicago in
1934 are shown copying
inscriptions in the
mastaba tomb of
Mereruka (ca. 2400
B.C.).

If, as many later commentators assumed, circumcision was a health mea-sure—a surgery mainly aimed at disease—it failed to find its way into the classic Egyptian medical texts. The magnificent papyri unearthed in the nine-teenth century by Edwin Smith and George Ebers make no mention of cir-cumcision. They do, however, reveal how Egyptians viewed the body, both as an object of science and a vessel of magical and divine forces.[4]

The Edwin Smith papyrus (ca. 1600 B.C.) is mainly a surgical manual, based on forty-eight detailed cases, advising the practitioner how to diagnose and treat fractures, wounds, and other injuries. "If thou examinest a man hav-ing a gaping wound in his shoulder," the writer advises,

> its flesh being laid back and its sides separated, while he suffers with swelling
> [in] his shoulder blade, thou shouldst palpate his wound. Shouldst thou find its
> gash separated from its sides in his wound, as a roll of linen is unrolled, [and] it
> is painful when he raises his arm on account of it, thou shouldst draw together
> for him his gash with stitching.[5]

The Smith papyrus has a great deal to say about wound dressings: plasters, poultices, cauteries, and purifying potions. Presumably the risks of circumcision were reduced because circumcised youths received careful postoperative treatment.

Just how far from the royal throne down into the social order the practice of circumcision reached is unknown. Some scholars have guessed that the procedure was limited to the elite: that in its early phase, circumcision was a mark of superior distinction reserved primarily for the priests, beginning with the pharaohs themselves, who were worshiped as the high priest of every god. In any case, however, it was not applied consistently. X-ray scans of Pharaoh Ahmose from the sixteenth century B.C. show that he died, a mature adult, uncircumcised. Elsewhere, ruins contain depictions of circumcised carpenters. The principle of selection remains elusive.[6]

Preventing excessive harm to the patient and producing a satisfactory aesthetic result took considerable skill. As in most circumcising cultures, the operation was performed by experts. Court physicians naturally stood atop the professional hierarchy; the circumcising priest of Saqqara may have been a physician as well. Whoever did the cutting did so in a public ceremony, and his job was to produce a noble, sacred wound. The surgery itself, dauntingly bloody and painful, was central to a temple ceremony rich with cultural overtones, for within the Egyptian city-states, temples were focal points of learning, medicine, and civil administration. They were seats of power, secular and divine.[7]

What did circumcision mean? Doubtless it was partly about purification. Purity was an Egyptian obsession, and one of medicine's main purposes was to purify, physically and spiritually. The Ebers papyrus suggests a deep-seated fear of contamination and putrefaction within the body. Enemas, purgatives, laxatives, along with all manner of cleaning compounds and disinfectants played a prominent role in the Egyptian medical armamentarium. (One of the few ancient healers whose name has survived was Iri, Keeper of the Royal Rectum, the pharaoh's gastroenterologist and colonic irrigation specialist.) Received wisdom held that the body's openings were portals through which not just impurities but malignant spirits might penetrate. Egyptian physiology took the Nile, with its channels and irrigation networks and its life-giving annual floods, as its controlling metaphor. Herodotus tells us that Egyptians spent three days a month purging their digestive tracts, certain that physical vitality, like the great river, depended on reliable flow.

This preoccupation with the body's excretions and secretions, and their bearing on health, is perhaps the best clue we have to why the Egyptians turned their attention to the foreskin. The foreskin harbors smegma. Particularly in hot climates, the space between the foreskin and the glans, unless washed regularly, can be a reservoir for malodorous secretions. Removing the foreskin may have been thought to cleanse the body's natural flow.

In the view of ancients who emulated the Egyptians, circumcision seems to have been not just a matter of hygiene but of moral, spiritual, and intellectual refinement. Origen, the influential biblical scholar and theologian of Alexandria, thought that Egyptians used circumcision to distinguish priests and intellectuals who committed themselves to the highest learning. "For among Egyptians," he wrote, "no one devoted himself to the study of astronomy, which was considered by them to be the noblest science, or at least to the secrets of astrology and genesis, which they considered to be the greatest thing, if he had not had himself circumcised." It was most likely his desire to purify himself, to subject the flesh to the nobler dictates of the spirit, that motivated Pythagoras, a devoted student of Egyptian wisdom, to have himself circumcised.

In the long sweep of history, Egypt first enshrined circumcision and accorded it a place of honor as a religious and social practice. Clearly the operation conferred exalted status. It became so important a symbol that over the centuries, members of Egypt's political, military, and commercial elites constantly pressured the priests to extend the mark to their sons. Hence circumcision became a mysterious object to which to aspire for the upper echelons of Egyptian society.

Yet ultimately it was in the religion of one of the Egyptians' subject peoples, the Israelites, that the ritual was established in the form that would become familiar in Judaism, Christianity, and Islam.

CIRCUMCISION AND JUDAISM

Though historically accurate, to say that ancient Israel inherited circumcision from Egypt vastly oversimplifies the complex relationship between two cultures. By the thirteenth century B.C., the age of Ramses II, circumcision had been established in Egypt for thousands of years. Certainly it was well known to Moses who led his people's escape from Egypt and began to put into place the main elements of law, ritual, and administrative authority essential to forming a Jewish nation. Historically, it was within this Mosaic religious paradigm that circumcision emerged as the characteristic mark of Judaism.

For all his tremendous authority and influence, Moses remains an almost ungraspable figure. By genealogy he is described as Israelite (Exodus 2), though from infancy he was adopted as a foundling into Pharaoh's court and raised among Egyptian royalty. The ambiguity of Moses' connection to the Israelites led some—most notoriously, Sigmund Freud—to conclude that he was in fact an Egyptian who, for reasons rooted deep within his own troubled psychology, took up the enslaved Hebrews' cause as his own.[8]

According to the biblical narrative, God commanded Moses to rescue the Israelites from captivity in Egypt and to reestablish the religion of Abraham and the former patriarchs, a religion whose defining ritual was circumcision. Moses was not circumcised while he lived in Pharaoh's household. Strangely enough, he would remain uncircumcised throughout his long life.

The oldest mention of circumcision in the Torah (not in biblical chronology, but in terms of the antiquity of the underlying source) is a cryptic account of a confrontation between Moses, God (Yahweh), and Zipporah, Moses' Midianite wife.

> Then it happened at a stopping place along the way that Yahweh met [Moses] and tried to kill him. Then Zipporah took a piece of flint and cut off her son's foreskin and touched [Moses'] feet with it, saying, "You are my blood-bridegroom." So [Yahweh] let him alone. At that time she said "blood-bridegroom" in reference to circumcision. (Exodus 4:24–26)

The sources of this extraordinary passage are extremely obscure. Understandably, it has provoked endless disputation among Jewish and Christian scholars concerned about reconciling it with the fuller picture of Moses and his relationship to God presented in the main narrative strands of the biblical text. Unusual elements include the baby's circumcision by his mother, the touching of the father's genitals ("feet") with the son's severed foreskin, and the magical transference of circumcision from Moses' infant son to the (uncircumcised) father. The phrase "blood-bridegroom" seems to echo a more primitive time in Israel's history when (as it remains in some tribes) circumcision may have been a premarriage initiation ritual, preparing the bridegroom's organ for procreation.

Though it is a cornerstone of Judaism, circumcision does not fit neatly into the biblical narrative. To begin with, Moses delivers a divine law that oddly he fails to exemplify. His lack of circumcision is just one among several prominent irregularities. Despite his heroic leadership, Moses is prevented from entering the land God promised to Israel and, unlike the patriarchs, is denied even the honor of being buried there. Some teachers within the rabbinic tradition interpreted this as God's punishment inflicted on Moses for not having been circumcised. As Rabbi Joshua Ben Karha said in the Mishna-Nedarim, "Great is the precept of circumcision for neglect of which Moses did not have his punishment suspended for even a single hour" (3:11). In any event he remains an enigma, a patriarch who, according to Old Testament scholar Peter Machinist, is in his "strangeness" a kind of antihero: someone who does not serve the native tradition at any point as a role model who can really be emulated."[9]

The man to be emulated, the Torah makes plain, is Abraham. With respect to the mythical lineage of Judaism, God revealed himself to Abraham, announcing that he and his descendants were to become God's chosen people. Biblical scholars have filled library shelves with analyses of place names, social practices, and archeological evidence in efforts to locate the "real" Abraham. Some have concluded, for example, that he lived in southern Mesopotamia sometime during the second millennium B.C. and headed a large seminomadic clan. But the fragmentary nature of the sources, beginning with the basic textual problems of the Torah itself, render such conclusions speculative at best. All we know of this patriarch of Judaism, Christianity, and Islam is the account set forth in the Book of Genesis.

Early in the process of developing religious self-consciousness, the community of ancient Israel came to believe that God had, in an ancient time, promised Abraham: "I will make of you a great nation." But this promise was conditional: it depended on Abraham's obedience, his observance of the covenant between them. According to the Genesis narrative, at the center of this covenant was circumcision, an outward symbol of Abraham's good faith.

> God said to Abraham, "For your part, you must keep my covenant, you and your descendants after you, generation by generation. This is how you shall keep my covenant between myself and you and your descendants after you: circumcise yourselves, every male among you. You shall circumcise the flesh of your foreskin, and it shall be the sign of the covenant between us. Every male among you in every generation shall be circumcised on the eighth day, both those born in your house and any foreigner, not of your blood but bought with your money. Circumcise both those born in your house and those bought with your money; thus shall my covenant be marked in your flesh as an everlasting covenant. (Genesis 17:10–13)

Most commentators within the Judeo-Christian and Muslim traditions, for whom Abraham is a seminal figure, have interpreted this passage literally. But even many who are not literalists have shared an underlying premise about Jewish exceptionalism. Scholars devoted to the history of ancient Israel have usually operated from an ingrained conviction that the religion of Israel, its theology and rituals, were essentially different from those of other people. The idea that strong ethnographic parallels existed between a primary ritual of Judaism and bloody rites of passage observed in primitive societies struck them as offensive to the point of being sacrilegious. Even if cutting the foreskin did arise in earlier times as a fertility ritual, wrote the distinguished historian Roland DeVaux, Israel's monotheistic "religion gave the rite a more lofty significance."[10]

Lofty yet also complicated. The Old Testament is not the product of a single author. It is a text composed of different narrative strands presenting distinctly different interpretations of God and the relationship between God and Israel. Compounding these textual problems, every event in the biblical narrative, every law and ritual, has for more than two millennia been subjected to layer upon layer of interpretation, first by Jewish priests and commentators, later by Christian scholars and theologians. Immense as this body of later commentary is, it sheds surprisingly little light on how ritual circumcision functioned in ancient Israel.

Language may offer the best clue to early meanings. Historical anthropologist Howard Eilberg-Schwartz points out that the Hebrew word characterizing the relationship between the covenant and circumcision is '*ôt*, meaning that the two are integrally related. Circumcision, in other words, was not merely a sign of the covenant; it constituted a vital part of the promise itself. In a sense circumcision literally *was* the covenant. This conception is reflected over many centuries, for rabbinical usage commonly referred to circumcision as "the covenant of our father Abraham." As feminist historian Gerda Lerner has remarked, "What is more logical and appropriate than to use as the leading symbol of the covenant the organ which produces this 'seed' and which 'plants' it in the female womb?"[11]

A covenant is a sacred agreement; in Abraham's case the agreement centered on a divine promise of miraculous fertility. Defining God's part of the bargain, God told Abraham:

> This is my covenant with you: You shall be the father of a multitude of nations. And you shall not longer be called Abram, but your name shall be Abraham, for I make you the father of a multitude of nations. I will make you exceedingly fertile, and make nations of you; and kings shall come forth from you. (Genesis 17:4–6)

Already very old, Abraham at first considered this promise risible, asking, "Can a child be born to a man a hundred years old, or can Sarah bear a child at ninety?" (Genesis 17:17). God's response, according to the narrative in Genesis, was to bless Abraham with fresh sexual vitality. Despite his age, he soon fathered a child, Isaac, with his wife Sarah. After Sarah died, he married a younger woman, Keturah, with whom he proceeded to produce a second family. Moreover, the fruits of the covenant were not limited to Abraham, for the promise encompassed his male offspring and slaves as well. Hence there is also a direct connection between circumcision and fertility in Abraham's circumcision of Ishmael, Abraham's son by Hagar, his wife's maid. Ishmael is sent away into the desert with his mother after the birth of Isaac. Nevertheless, Abraham wanted Ishmael, like himself, to be the father of multitudes. Because Ishmael is circumcised, God grants this wish even though Ishmael is otherwise excluded from the promise of the Abrahamic covenant. On this score, Eilberg-Schwartz notes, "Ishmael's circumcision would make no sense at all if circumcision was only a sign of the covenant."[12]

Along with its promise, God's speech to Abraham includes a threat. "Every uncircumcised male, everyone who has not had the flesh of his foreskin circumcised, shall be cut off from his people. He has broken my covenant" (Genesis 17:14). On its face, this seems to mean that the uncircumcised—those who do not bear the tribal sign—are to be ostracized from the community. Among a desert-dwelling tribe who monopolized a region's scarce resources of food and water, such banishment amounted to a death sentence. In addition, as some medieval commentators observed, "cut off from his people" may also mean that the uncircumcised would suffer the curse of infertility or impotence, almost as serious a threat as expulsion. Inability to produce descendants was, to a staunchly patriarchal people, bitterly disgraceful.[13]

Because circumcision was applied to all males, Jewish writers came to think of removing the foreskin as normal. Tradition taught that beyond symbolizing Israel's covenant with God, circumcision prepared the penis to function as God intended. To this way of thinking, circumcision was natural and healthy. Thus it followed that being uncircumcised connoted physical or spiritual debility. Moses, for example, who evidently suffered a speech impediment, is twice described in the Torah as being afflicted with uncircumcised lips. More generally, *uncircumcised* is used as a metonym to slur the Philistines (I Samuel 18:25), suggesting that because they were not party to the covenant with God, they constituted a lower order of being.

Biblical writers discussed circumcision more frequently as a metaphor than as a physical fact. A characteristic passage in Deuteronomy urges the person who resists God, "Circumcise therefore the foreskin of your heart, and be no more stiff-necked" (Deuteronomy 10:16). Elsewhere, circumcision of the heart is described as a divine act, a kind of spiritual surgery: "And the Lord your God will circumcise your heart, and the heart of your offspring, to love the Lord your God with all your heart, and with all your soul, that you may live" (Deuteronomy 30:6). Later the prophet Jeremiah uses the same phrase, exploiting the distinction between nominal circumcision (of the foreskin) and true circumcision (of the heart). "The time shall come when I will punish all the circumcised that are uncircumcised," Jeremiah inveighs on behalf of the Lord. "For all the nations are uncircumcised, but Israel is uncircumcised at heart" (Jeremiah 9:25–26). He adds that those who have failed to heed God's words have uncircumcised ears.

Circumcision constituted a strong metaphor for submission to the divine will, and Old Testament writers did not limit it to the human body. Among the point-by-point dietary laws set forth in Leviticus we find the following passage:

When you enter the land and plant any tree for food, you shall regard its fruit as its foreskin. Three years it shall be uncircumcised for you, not to be eaten. In the fourth year all its fruit shall be set aside for jubilation before the Lord; and only in the fifth year may you use its fruit—that its yield to you may be increased: I am the Lord your God. (Leviticus 19:23–25)[14]

The fruit trees growing in Israel—figs, olives, grapes, dates, and so forth—typically produce very little fruit during their early years. Their capacity to bear fruit comes only with maturity. In this respect, the writer suggests, they resemble the uncircumcised child, whose fertility awaits the removal of his foreskin in preparation for sexual intercourse and fathering offspring. Eilberg-Schwartz surmises that the authors of Leviticus were drawing an analogy between excising the foreskin and pruning trees. Trimming was meant to increase fecundity. "Both acts of cutting remove unwanted excess and both increase the desired yield," he writes. "One might say that when Israelites circumcise their male children, they are pruning the fruit trees of God."[15]

Despite the signal importance of circumcision, the Old Testament is notably vague about its details. In the days of Moses and his followers, the Jewish pilgrims apparently circumcised at puberty or early adulthood. As with the Egyptians, the instrument of choice was a stone blade. Shortly after Joshua led the Israelites across the river Jordan, according to the biblical narrative, the Lord commanded him, "Make yourself flint knives and squat down and circumcise the people of Israel for a second time. So Joshua made flint knives and circumcised the people of Israel on the hill of foreskins" (Joshua 5:2–3). Clearly the people circumcised in this group ritual were not infants but, as in Egypt, adolescents or older males. (The squatting position itself is reminiscent of Egyptian practice.) In the view of many anthropologists, fashioning a blade from flint indicates a sense of connection with the earth and its elements, blood mingled with stone, which is characteristic of tribal circumcision rites around the world and throughout history. Allusion to the hill of foreskins— evidently a place historically connected with the ritual—reinforces the idea that in Israel's early phases, circumcision involved the collective spilling of blood among one's kin. Anthropologist Max Gluckman characterized this as a type of blood brotherhood.[16]

The Old Testament is full of violence, and circumcision is frequently identified with brutality, occasionally with death. In one episode, to avenge the rape of their sister Dinah by a Hivite named Shechem (who subsequently proposed to marry her) Jacob's sons tell the young prince, "We cannot give our sister to a man who is uncircumcised; for we look upon that as a disgrace." The scheme of revenge they devise is for the prince, along with all the men in his tribe, to submit themselves to circumcision, based on the promise that afterward the two families and communities will be able to intermarry. The Hivites foolishly agree. "Every one of them was circumcised, every able-bodied male. Then two days later, when they were in great pain, Jacob's two sons Simeon and Levi, full brothers to Dinah, armed themselves with swords, boldly entered the city and killed every male" (Genesis 34:1–25).

In another grisly incident, King Saul, as a condition of allowing David to marry his daughter, demands an unusual dowry: "All the king wants as the bride-price is the foreskins of a hundred Philistines, by way of vengeance on his enemies." Saul considers this a clever way to get rid of a potential rival. But David and his band, to prove their mettle, proceed to double Saul's quota, slaughtering two hundred Philistines. David "brought their foreskins and counted them out to the king in order to be accepted as his son-in-law" (I Samuel 18:24–29). Though the text reads "foreskins," this is probably misleading because Old Testament writers refrained from explicitly naming the penis. David in all likelihood did not posthumously circumcise his slain enemies but rather, in a practice common to many tribes, cut off their genitals as trophies of conquest.

At some point Israelite circumcision was transformed into a neonatal operation. In ancient Egypt, as in most tribal societies that practice the ritual, it served as a rite of passage, part of a ceremony whose themes include fertility, intergenerational continuity, and the transition from boyhood to sexual and social maturity. Against this pattern, the Israelite circumcision of babies on the eighth day of life seems exceptional, closely associated not with marriage but with birth.

Pondering the question of why his forebears established *infant* circumcision, Philo Judaeus, a Hellenistic Jewish philosopher writing in Alexandria, decided it had to do with confirming the child's commitment to the community before he had any choice in the matter. "It is very much better and more farsighted of us to prescribe circumcision for infants," he said, "for perhaps one who is full-grown would hesitate through fear to carry out this ordinance of his own free will."[17] Philo, who constantly struggled to discover rational explanations for Jewish law and practice, associated circumcision with fertility, along with other benefits. The uncircumcised foreskin, he wrote, may prevent semen from making its way into the vagina. Therefore, "such nations as practise circumcision increase greatly in population." Anticipating Eilberg-Schwartz, Philo saw an analogy between circumcising "home-born and purchased" boys and pruning trees. "There is need for both of these to be purified and trimmed like plants . . . for well-grown [plants] produce many superfluous [fruits] because of the fertility, which it is useful to cut off." Oddly, however, even though he thought it promoted fertility, Philo held that circumcision blunted sexual sensation. "The legislators thought good to dock the organ which ministers to such intercourse," he wrote, introducing a theme that would become prominent in the Middle Ages, "thus making circumcision the symbol of excision of excessive and superfluous pleasure."[18]

Infant circumcision reflected both faith in the covenant and the desire to distinguish Israelite males from their uncircumcised neighbors, a concern that grew acute during the Babylonian exile (587–522 B.C.). In the minds of the priests, the permanence of the mark bestowed in infancy was important to keep Jews from deserting their community. Indeed, the procedure itself became more radical, removing a larger portion of the foreskin in order to ensure that those who were circumcised as infants would be unable to evade their Jewish identity.

They had ample motives for evasion. After Alexander the Great conquered the Near East between 334 and 331 B.C., a vogue of Greek culture inaugurated by Alexander himself and sustained by his followers swept through Jewish communities. Circumcision, as a mutilation of the natural human form, violated Greek esthetics. Moreover, Greeks held athletic contests in which participants appeared nude. The Greek standard of modesty held that the fore-skin should cover the glans. Visible glans in an uncircumcised man was taken as evidence of sexual arousal and was thus considered indecent within the arena. To prevent mishaps, many athletes wore the *kynodesme*, a strand of col-ored string that looped around the foreskin, closing it tightly over the glans. The Greek code of genital etiquette placed circumcised Jews at an embarrass-ing disadvantage in the public baths, wrestling matches, and competitive games. To compensate, as the Maccabean report noted around 100 B.C., Jew-ish athletes "constructed a Gentile-style gymnasium in Jerusalem. They also pulled forward their prepuces thereby repudiating the holy covenant" (I Mac-cabees 1:15). The desire of young men to appear uncircumcised was a source of continuing annoyance to the priests. Josephus, the eminent Jewish histo-rian, commented on the trend among Jews in the first century. "They also hid the circumcision of their genitals, that even when they were naked they might appear to be Greeks."

This was not merely a desire to fit in. Josephus remarked on Gentile hos-tility to circumcision. Many Jewish men who sought to disguise or reverse their circumcisions were reacting to a pervasive Greco-Roman antipathy, an aversion that historian Peter Schäfer describes as "the deeply felt threat that the Jewish superstition might succeed in finally destroying the cultural and re-ligious values of Roman society."[19] First-century biographer and historian Suetonious, who had once served as Hadrian's secretary, recalled that

> in the days of Domitian the collection of the Jewish tax was carried out with
> especial severity. . . . I myself remember a scene from my youth, when the
> Procurator, surrounded by a host of his assistants, subjected an old man of
> about ninety to a physical examination, in order to determine whether or not
> he was circumcised.[20]

Philo conveys a sense of contemporary attitudes at the opening of his *Special Laws*:

> I will begin with that which is an object of ridicule among many people. Now
> the practice which is thus ridiculed, namely the circumcision of the genital or-
> gans, is very zealously observed by many other nations . . . . And therefore it
> would be well for the detractors to desist from childish mockery and to inquire
> in a wise and more serious spirit into the causes to which the performance of
> this custom is due, instead of dismissing the matter prematurely and impugn-
> ing the good sense of great nations. (*Special Laws*, 1.2–1.3)

In part, such derision stemmed from confusion between circumcision and castration. Most people outside Judaism, for whom the foreskin and penis were not sharply distinguished, had no idea exactly what cutting was performed on Jewish babies' genitals. Circumcision was among the mysteries of an alien religion, subject to much misunderstanding and rumor. A passage from *Pesiqta de Rab Kahana*, a collection of traditional Jewish legends about Israel in biblical times that reflects attitudes of the Romans during the era of Hadrian, shows how circumcision could be interpreted as bizarre mutilation, deserving contempt.

> Just what did the retinue of Amalek use to do? They would cut off the circumcised organ of generation from live Israelites and would fling it heavenwards, taunting God: 'Is this what you have chosen? Here is what you chose for yourself.'[21]

In contrast, the rabbis defended circumcision by arguing that the foreskin was an imperfection whose removal was necessary to reveal the body's ideal form. "In the case of a fig, its only defect is its stalk," taught one prominent rabbi. "Remove it and blemish ceases. Thus, the Holy One Blessed be He said to Abraham, 'Your only defect is this foreskin. Remove it and the blemish is cancelled. Walk before Me and be perfect.' "[22]

The Tannaim (teachers who transmitted sacred oral tradition in the first and second centuries) told stories of how Jews cleverly, sometimes heroically, preserved their ritual in the face of persecution. According to one account, a Jewish wise man approached the Roman leaders, who had banned circumcision on grounds that it was harmful to health and vitality, and posed the following question: "If one has an enemy, what does he with him, to be weak or healthy?" The Romans naturally answered, "Weak." Whereupon the Tanna sage countered, "Then let their children be circumcised at the age of eight days and they will be weak." Unable to resist this logic, the story goes, the Romans conceded, "He speaks rightly," and reversed the ban.

During cycles of bitter repression and struggles for control over Jewish peoples and lands, circumcision became a matter of life and death. Antiochus Epiphanes, the draconian ruler of Judea during the second century B.C., imposed severe penalties for circumcision as part of his assault on Judaism (I Maccabees 1:48 and 2 Maccabees 6:10). *Mohels* who performed the ritual could be crucified, stoned, or fed to wild dogs. Mothers who permitted the circumcision of their babies "were garroted, their strangled infants strung

about their necks, then hanged upon crosses as a terrible warning to others."
Alternatively, when John Hyrcanus I, political leader and high priest of Israel,
consolidated his control over the country and pulled down the Samaritan
temple on Mt. Gerizim, he proceeded to force Judaism—and circumcision—
upon all the people of southern Judea.[23]

It was from this group, called the Idumeans, that Herod the Great arose.
His Jewish ancestry ambiguous, Herod sought to ratify his heritage through
circumcision. Josephus tells how, in order to confirm his identity with the Jews
and thus his authority to rule Judea, Herod forced a young man named
Sylleus, the Arabian suitor of his sister Salome, to submit to circumcision as a
condition of marriage. Two generations later, Herod's grandson Agrippa, diffi-
dent about his own Jewish identity, followed his grandfather's example, agreeing to give his daughter's hand in marriage to a foreign sovereign only on the
condition that the king have himself circumcised.[24]

Faced with tyrannical oppression, some Jews sought permanently to erase
evidence of circumcision, using surgical means to recreate a foreskin. During
the period of persecutions that culminated with the disastrous Judean revolt
against Rome led by Bar Koziba in 132 C.E., operations to reverse circumcision were widespread. The most common technique was a painful and tedious
process the Greeks called *epispasmos*. Stretching out whatever skin remained of
the prepuce, "they tie and draw together the skin [over] the glans, making it
tight all around with glue, thus renewing the prepuce." If only a portion of the
foreskin had been excised, the stretching and binding was fairly easy. The
Greek word for such men was *epispastics*, meaning "to draw in" the foreskin.
Their status within Judaism has been ambiguous. For example, the *Midrash
Tanchuma*, in its rabbinic commentary on the Book of Genesis, suggests that
Esau was an epispastic.

A more extreme option was the knife. "If the glans is bare," wrote first-
century master surgeon Aurelius Cornelius Celsus, "and a man decides for de-
cency's sake to cover it, this may be accomplished." As described in Celsus'
celebrated work, *De Medicina*, uncircumcision involved cutting away the connective tissue between the glans and remaining foreskin, then in effect turning the prepuce inside out and pulling the exposed tissue toward the tip of the
glans. Patients undergoing this painful procedure no doubt would have been
thankful for the opium poppies Celsus prescribed. To prevent the stretched
foreskin from shrinking back to a retracted position, he advised bandaging the
penis from the root to the tip of the glans, and plastering the raw preputial
skin with healing salve.[25]

Alarmed that men were using modern medical arts to abandon their religion, rabbis solemnly predicted the dire consequences of such procedures. "Great is the importance of the fulfillment of the covenant connected with the circumcision," a distinguished commentator said, "that if one who is circumcised has in mind to render himself by artificial devices uncircumcised, he has no share in the world to come." To discourage men from trying to restore their foreskins, the traditional operation was revised. *Milah*, as the first state of circumcision is called, simply meant cutting off a portion of an infant's foreskin. Still, enough of it usually remained to enable a surgeon to create something resembling an uncircumcised penis. To prevent this, probably around the middle of the second century, rabbis augmented *milah* with *periah*, a radical ablation of the foreskin that bared the glans entirely. Once established, *periah* was deemed essential to circumcision; if the *mohel* failed to cut away enough tissue, the operation was deemed insufficient to comply with God's covenant. Depending on the strictness of individual rabbis, boys (or men thought to have been inadequately cut) were subjected to additional operations. "The tender covering under the skin is to be rent with the nails," declared the authoritative Joreh Deah. "Circumcision without tearing is the equivalent of no circumcision at all.[26]

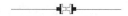

In the Christian era, many intellectual and spiritual traditions in Judaism carried circumcision far beyond its biblical origins. If there is a single dominant theme in the rabbinic texts that elucidated the rite for successive generations, it was a growing emphasis on blood. To cite one example, the classic ritual included naming the eight-day-old boy, and the naming prayer in *berit milah* borrows a passage from the Book of Ezekiel: "And it is said, 'I passed by you and saw you wallowing in your blood, and I said to you: "In your blood, live" ' " (Ezekiel 16:6). Interpreting this, Rabbi Eliezar wrote, "it must be that God said, 'By merit of the blood of covenantal circumcision and the blood of the paschal lamb I will redeem you from Egypt. On account of their merit you will be saved at the end of days.' "[27]

Historian Lawrence Hoffman illustrates that, in this and many other sources, circumcision blood is elevated to supreme importance. "The Rabbis replaced the fertility symbolism of the Bible with blood as a symbol of salvation," he wrote. "In this blood symbolism, they merged the two biblical concepts of covenant—sacrifice (from Genesis 15) and circumcision (from

Genesis 17)." One reads in *Seder Rav Amram Gaon*, a prayer book published in the ninth century, the following:

> They bring water containing myrtle and various very sweet-smelling spices, and they circumcise the child so that the blood of the circumcision falls into the water. Then all the designated people wash their hands in it, as if to say, 'This is the blood of circumcision that mediates between God and Abraham our father.'

The practice of mixing circumcision blood and water was not limited to one time or to one group. Contrasting Jewish rituals in different countries, one medieval text noted that whereas "in the Land of Israel, they circumcise over earth . . . in Babylonia, they circumcise over water, and put it on their faces."[28]

In the rabbinic imagination, the blood of the paschal lamb, commemorating God's deliverance of Israel from bondage in Egypt, and the blood of circumcision, symbolizing God's covenant with Abraham and his descendants, flowed together. Understanding this helps us grasp the profound significance of wine in seder and circumcision as a symbol of blood that saves: the blood of a male lamb at Passover, the blood of a male infant at *berit milah.*

Modern scholars have noticed a basic gender bias in the distinction between circumcision blood and the blood flowing from women in menses and childbirth. Israel was intensely patriarchal. Traditionally, women were assigned marginal roles in Jewish religious life, a marginalization reinforced by their exclusion from circumcision, the central mark of God's covenant. And while circumcision blood grew holier through the centuries, the rabbis, citing explicit taboos dictated in the Book of Leviticus (15:19–30), painted a picture of vaginal blood as uncontrolled, impure, and dangerous. Male blood was about salvation, female about pollution. So great was the bias that women were occasionally excluded from the *berit milah* ceremony. There is no evidence that before modern times rabbinic Judaism ever considered a covenant ritual for females. For most of Jewish history, a woman's title to the covenant was derivative, its central symbol reserved for husbands and sons.[29]

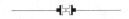

What did salvation mean? The Talmud teaches how circumcision is to figure in the Jewish afterlife:

In the Hereafter Abraham will sit at the entrance of *Gehinnom* [Hell] and will not allow any circumcised Israelite to descend into it. As for those who sinned unduly, what does he do to them? He removes the foreskin from children who had died before circumcision, places it upon them and sends them down to *Gehinnom*.

Rabbi Eliezar agreed, declaring, "He who makes void the Covenant of Abraham our Father has not position in the World to Come."[30]

The Midrash, an expansive genre of rabbinic interpretation and exposition of scriptural texts, comments at length on the import of circumcision. We learn in the Midrash-Nedarim, for example, that "circumcision is great since, but for that, the Holy one would not have created his world" (3:11). This follows from a rather far-fetched interpretation of a single passage in the Book of Jeremiah, in which God says: "But for my covenant by day and night I would not have set forth the ordinances of Heaven and earth" (Jeremiah 34:27). Elsewhere, stories abound about patriarchs, from Adam to Job, who were born circumcised.

So too the Kabbalah, a body of mystical teachings and secret doctrines, purports to fathom the ritual's deeper mysteries. The Kabbalah's principle text is the Zohar, traditionally believed to embody the teachings of Rabbi Simeon bar Yochai and his followers, who dwelt in Palestine during the second and third centuries A.D. In its approach to circumcision, the Zohar places special emphasis on themes of sacrifice and the importance of shedding blood. Here, for example, is Rabbi Abba's interpretation of the mystical meaning of God's promise, "Your people shall be righteous" (Isaiah 60:21):

Happy are Israel who bring an offering willingly to the Holy One, blessed be He, for they bring their sons on the eighth day as an offering. And when they are circumcised they enter into a goodly portion of the Holy One, blessed be He, as it is written, "The righteous is the foundation of the world" [Proverbs 10:25].

Elsewhere, Rabbi Simeon remarks that in circumcision, "the blood that comes from the child is preserved before the Holy One, Blessed be He. And when judgments are aroused in the world, the Holy One, blessed be He, looks at the blood, and saves the world."[31]

In later centuries, the most thoughtful and articulate of Jewish commentators who dealt with the question of circumcision was Moses Maimonides, the great philosophical and legal genius of the Jewish Middle Ages. Born in Spain in 1135, trained in medicine and schooled in philosophy, Maimonides moved to Cairo where he became personal physician to Saladin. His magnum opus, *Guide to the Perplexed*, remains a classic effort to balance faith and reason. Because the physician in him knew that cutting a baby's penis seemed illogical and risky, Maimonides devoted particular attention to developing a rationale for circumcision.

"No one," he insisted, "should circumcise himself or his son for any other reason than pure faith." This conceded, he moved on to argue that circumcision in itself was an utterly indispensable part of Jewish law, and that the operation on the penis had a beneficial effect on a man, making it easier for him to obey the rest of the law. The overarching purpose of the law, he wrote, was "to quell all the impulses of matter."[32] Extraordinary mutual love and communal bonds flowed from circumcision, because the mark—a physical token men shared—not only linked them in the flesh but constantly reminded them of their higher spiritual unity as descendants of Abraham and heirs to the covenant. Outwardly, he wrote, it united "those who believe in the unity of God," enabling Jews to recognize each other and not fall prey to strangers. Counterfeits were unthinkable. No man would willingly choose such an operation for himself unless it was the result of the deepest conviction, for "it is a very, very hard thing."

Indeed, fear and pain were the reasons that the operation was best performed on newborns. Maimonides acknowledged that unless circumcision was performed in early infancy, Jews were likely to ignore the law. Few men would willingly submit to an excruciating ordeal. Like most physicians throughout history, Maimonides assumed that infants felt less pain from the operation than older children or men. A baby's "membrane is still soft and his imagination weak," he said. Whereas a grown man would become sick with dread simply thinking about the operation beforehand, an infant, he felt sure, would experience no apprehension and would quickly forget the pain. Parents also had less anxiety about an early circumcision. With a newborn, Maimonides said, parents' love was also nascent, making it far easier for them to cut their child than it would be later when their love and empathy were fully formed.[33]

Although Maimonides thought that parents could tolerate circumcision only if they disregarded the distress it caused their sons, he was at the same time convinced that "the bodily pain caused to [the penis] is the real purpose of circumcision." The blood, the discomfort, the violent excision of the skin covering of the male organ—this early trauma, he concluded, permanently weakened a man's sexual appetite and dulled the pleasure he derived from sexual intercourse. "With regard to circumcision, one of the reasons for it is, in my opinion, the wish to bring about a decrease in sexual intercourse and a weakening of the organ in question, so that this activity be diminished and the organ be in as quiet a state as possible." By suppressing a potential source of fleshly temptation, the argument went, circumcision promoted spirituality. The sages knew that the foreskin heightened sexual experience, Maimonides said, just as it was common knowledge that "it is hard for a woman with whom an uncircumcised man has had sexual intercourse to separate from him."* By reducing sensuality, making intercourse less pleasurable and more practical, it helped lessen men's obsession with sex. Circumcision served most of the spiritual purposes of castration without depriving a man of his fertility.[34]

Maimonides recognized an implicit contradiction in this view. If a man were better off without the foreskin, why had God created it in the first place? "How can natural things be defective so they need to be corrected from outside," he asked, "all the more so because we know how useful the foreskin is for that member?" His answer, a weak one, was that circumcision was not actually a physical correction but a moral or psychological one. "Moral qualities of the soul are consequent on the temperament of the body," he said, and the law, driven into the recalcitrant body by the intellect, was God's mechanism for subduing the flesh. In this respect, his theory was consistent with the Midrash Tadshe, which proclaimed the medieval belief that "the covenant of circumcision was therefore placed on the genitals so that the fear of God would restrain them from sin."[35]

An offshoot of Maimonides' theory was the notion that circumcision protects Jews from destructive sexual urges. A thirteenth-century French commentator and follower of Maimonides, Isaac ben Yediah, expounded at length with surprising erotic explicitness about the "advantages" the Jew enjoyed over the uncircumcised Christian. When a beautiful woman makes love to an uncircumcised man, he wrote,

---

*The notion that circumcision depressed sexual drive was widely shared. What had been a sign of blessing under the old covenant could be interpreted as a mark of weakness under the new. Gabriello Fallopio, one of the great anatomists of the Italian Renaissance, contended that the foreskin made sexual intercourse more pleasurable. Accordingly, God must have imposed circumcision so that Abraham and his progeny would concentrate on serving Him rather than pursuing the pleasures of the flesh.

she feels pleasure and reaches an orgasm first. When an uncircumcised man sleeps with her and then resolves to return to his home, she brazenly grasps him, holding onto his genitals and says to him, "come back, make love to me." This is because of the pleasure that she finds in intercourse with him, from the sinews of his testicles—sinew of iron—and from his ejaculation—that of a horse—which he shoots like an arrow into her womb.

The couple makes love two and three times a night, day after day, "yet the appetite is not filled."

With the Jew, owing to his circumcision, sex is a different story. "He will find himself performing his task quickly, emitting his seed as soon as he inserts the crown. . . . As soon as he begins intercourse with [his wife], he immediately comes to a climax." For her part, the woman "has no pleasure from him." She leaves the marriage bed aroused and frustrated. "She does not have an orgasm once a year, except on rare occasions, because of the great heat and fire burning in her." But the husband can take heart, Isaac concluded, because, freed from his lascivious desires, he "will not empty his brain because of his wife [and] his heart will be strong to seek out God."[36]

In the eighteenth century, certain Hasidic ascetics would go even further, suggesting that circumcision converted the pleasure of sexual intercourse into pain. "Copulation is difficult for the true zaddik," Naham of Bratslav admonished his followers. "Not only does he have no desire for it at all, but he experiences real suffering in the act, suffering which is like that which the infant undergoes when he is circumcised. The very same suffering, to an even greater degree, is felt by the zaddik during intercourse."[37]

Because he invested it with such great importance and as a physician understood the anatomy of the operation better than most, Maimonides offered technical advice on performing the physical procedure.

> The entire foreskin, which covers the glans, is cut, so that the whole of the glans is exposed. Then the thin layer of skin beneath the foreskin is divided with the nail and turned back, till the flesh of the glans is completely exposed. The wound is then sucked till the blood has been drawn from parts remote from the surface thus obviating danger to the child. After this has been done, a plaster, bandage, or similar dressing is applied.

He also covered unusual cases and rare medical conditions. If a male infant was born without a foreskin, the child must nonetheless go through the traditional ceremony on the eighth day, with the *mohel* using his blade to scratch the child's penis to draw blood. Babies with ambiguous genitalia, including hermaphrodites and those born with two penises, were to be circumcised as well. Children born prematurely or with manifest symptoms of disease presented a different problem. Sick infants were not to be circumcised until they recovered, and if the illness were systemic (e.g., jaundice) there was to be a seven-day waiting period to ensure recovery was complete.

Hemophilia, a genetic abnormality that interferes with blood clotting, though poorly understood, was a matter of grave concern. Cutting a hemophiliac baby could cause uncontrollable hemorrhage and death. Unfortunately, until the twentieth century, there was no sure way of diagnosing the disorder in advance. Talmudic wisdom decreed that if two male children died from bleeding after circumcision, the third son should be spared the ritual. The exception for bleeding disorders meant that there was, throughout the past several centuries, a minority of Jews who were exempted from circumcision for medical reasons.[38] Maimonides, who considered circumcision a matter of critical importance, suggested that even if two brothers had died, a third boy might be circumcised after infancy, once "his strength is established." To his way of thinking, "one may only circumcise a child that is totally free from disease because danger to life overrides every other consideration. It is possible to circumcise later than the proper time, but it is impossible to restore a single departed soul of Israel forever." Along these lines, the Talmud relates the following narrative of a Jewish teacher.

On one occasion, I went to the land of Kaputkia, and a woman came before me who had her first son circumcised and he died and her second son circumcised and he died. The third [son] she brought before me. I saw that he was green [with anemia] and I examined him and saw no covenant blood in him. I told her to wait until he become full-blooded. She waited and then had him circumcised, and he lived and he was called by the name Nathan the Babylonian after my name.[39]

Gradually the rabbinical tradition came to understand that bleeding disorders were hereditary. As Joseph Caro wrote in the sixteenth century, "there are families in which the blood is loose." In modern practice, a child diagnosed with hemophilia is exempt from circumcision. A laboratory test confirming that his blood lacks a clotting factor has replaced the deaths of two siblings as sufficient evidence of disease.[40]

The Shulchan Aruch, the standard reference for Jewish ritual observance, notes that for all its symbolic meaning, circumcision does not make a boy a Jew. The uncircumcised Jew remains, by virtue of birth, a member of the Jewish community. Still, the *berit milah* (covenant of circumcision) or bris (from the Hebrew word for covenant) has remained a central ritual within Judaism, a sacred obligation, an affirmation of one's Jewish heritage. "Circumcision draws down a level of Divine light which the Jews cannot draw down through their Divine service," one Mishnah commentator observed. "The act of circumcision is necessary, because as long as the foreskin is present, the light will not be drawn down. It is only when the foreskin is removed that the light will reveal itself."[41]

The bris is scheduled during the daylight hours of the eighth day of life, no matter whether that day falls on the Sabbath or a religious holiday. Indeed, early rabbis agreed, as Rabbi Jose said in the Mishna-Nedarim, "Circumcision is a great precept for it overrides the strictness of the Sabbath." Sometimes it may be postponed: if the child was delivered via caesarean section, if the *mohel* is not within walking distance, if the baby is sickly or weighs less than five pounds. Nowadays, the ceremony typically takes twenty minutes. The baby's mother lights candles (with no blessing said). The baby is carried into the room on a pillow. The *mohel* explains the meaning of the procedure, noting that entering one's child into the covenant of circumcision affirms his sacred obligation to improve the world. The infant is placed on the Chair of Elijah, symbolizing the prayer that the baby lives his life in a world of peace and righteousness. (The rabbis considered Elijah the patron of circumcision, his spirit always present at each ceremony.) It is an honor to convey the baby into the room and to place him on the chair, but the most honored person is the *Sandik*, who holds the baby while the foreskin is cut and when the child is given his Jewish name. Afterward, those assembled join in a meal of celebration.[42]

Rabbis worked out a system for dealing with boys who are adopted or converted to Judaism. An infant not born to a Jewish mother may have a bris on any day except the Sabbath or a Jewish holiday. An infant circumcised at birth in the hospital or an older boy who is already circumcised must undergo token circumcision. This is a procedure known as *Hatafat Dam Berit* (drawing the blood of the covenant), in which the *mohel* punctures the penis with a lancet, just enough to draw blood. It is performed on male candidates for conversion of any age; all converts to Judaism must be circumcised. After the age of six months, in countries with modern health care facilities, the operation is performed in a hospital, with a *mohel* present in the operating room.

For the better part of two thousand years, Jewish circumcision followed a three-step pattern. First was *chituch*, the cutting of the stretched foreskin. Then came *periah*, the complete exposure of the glans of the penis effected by cutting or tearing away all the inner foreskin tissue back to the frenulum. Finally, with the operation finished, came *mezizah*, a practice in which the *mohel* sucked the blood from the wounded penis until the bleeding stopped. Ethnographer Felix Bryk captured the classic technique of the *mohel* at work in the following passage.

> He takes the member by the thumb and forefinger of his left and rubs it several times gently to evoke an erection; he then takes hold of the outer and inner lamellae of the foreskin on both sides . . . and draws them down over the glans, pressing them smooth, by lifting his hand upward at the same time and thus giving the member a vertical position. The *mohel* now takes a pair of small pincers in the thumb and forefinger of his right hand and inserts the foreskin into the crack in such a manner than the glans comes to be behind it and the foreskin that is to be cut away in front of it. Then he takes hold of the knife with the first three fingers of his right hand in such a manner that it rests on the middle finger, with the index finger on the back of the knife and the thumb on the handle. With one vertical motion downwards he cuts off close to the plate the part of the foreskin that is before it, which is being held with the left hand. If this has been done according to prescription . . . the foreskin itself is clipped at the tip, resulting in an opening about the size of a pea.[43]

The surgery was not finished. To accomplish *periah* and complete the denudation of the glans, the *mohel* set aside his instruments and used only his thumbnail, long, lancet-shaped, filed to the sharpest possible edge. (In the closing decades of the nineteenth century, European and American circumcisers gradually took up scissors and other surgical instruments, though many of them continued to wear the distinctive nail.)

> Directly after the cut has been made, the *mohel* puts the tip of his thumb nail . . . into the opening of the inner lamella of the foreskin, grasps the foreskin by its tip with the help of both index fingers, splits it on the back of the glans by means of slitting up to the crown of the latter, and shoves the slit foreskin up over the crown of the glans.[44]

The incisions completed, the *mohel* pinched the foreskin between his thumb and index finger and tore it away from the penis.

Mezizah b'peh followed immediately, the *mohel* taking the bleeding penis in his mouth, sucking the blood, then turning to take mouthfuls of wine from a goblet and spitting this wine on the infant's wound. He laid that foreskin in a small basin of sand that had earlier been placed near the child. Then, pouring a fresh goblet of wine, he proclaimed a blessing and offered a brief prayer. By this time the bleeding had stopped, and the baby needed only a simple linen bandage.

As the sole rite of initiation of a newborn male into the community, circumcision underwent substantial changes between late antiquity, when it was a domestic event, and the Middle Ages, when it expanded to include the wider community and into the synagogue. Symbolism in the ceremony became richer. Historian Ivan Marcus tells us, for example, that the Chair of Elijah was introduced to the circumcision ritual and to the seder to connect these rituals to Israel's prophetic past and messianic future. At both ceremonies the empty chair awaits the prophet whose arrival is the harbinger of the coming of the messiah and the fulfillment of God's covenant with Israel. Thus circumcision came to be associated with a "symbol of messianic days to be enjoyed by the entire Jewish people . . . thereby placing a onetime event in the life of a particular child into a cosmic framework."[45]

Even as its spiritual significance grew more communal during this period, circumcision presented an opportunity for popular celebration, blending elements of the sacred and the profane. In Palestine, the occasion of circumcision itself had long been an occasion of feasting and rejoicing. "My father, Abayah, was one of the notable men of his generation, and at my circumcision he invited all the notables of Jerusalem," one reads in Midrash Rabbah Ruth. "And when they had eaten and drunk, they sang some ordinary songs and others alphabetized acrostics" (6:4). In Central Europe and Italy, beginning in the Middle Ages, the nights before a boy's circumcision became a time of extended revelry. "Festival jollity and facetious merriment," were the words Johannes Buxtorf, a Swiss Hebraist in the early seventeenth century, used to describe *Wachnact*. Ostensibly the gathering was supposed to comfort the child's mother, warding off her fears of the surgery and protecting mother and child from evil spirits. Buxtorf scoffed, however, that *Wachnacht* was really just an excuse to paint the town. Men and women stuffed themselves with bread and meat and consumed copious amounts of alcohol. If a few prayers were said for the child, they were drowned out by the unruly gambling, singing, and dancing that often carried on until dawn.[46] The partying was equally raucous in Italy. In 1727, the rabbi of Rome's Jewish community wrote:

The custom is that when a man has a male child born to him . . . tumultuous sounds rise forth from his home throughout the night before the circumcision. For the father gathers together his friends and relatives . . . to display the pomp and splendor of his majesty . . . and with a joyous heart they partake of delicacies . . . in accord with their desire, in a matter worse than their father. They drink fine wine from elegant vessels . . . and instead of reciting prayers of praise and thanksgiving to God, all sing lusty sounds with their faces ablaze. They engage in vain and ridiculous activities, young and old, women and children. Some dance, young men and maidens together, mouthing obscenities and devising sins in their hearts, while others give utterance to the evil desires of their souls, drinking to forget their abject poverty.[47]

Such partying infuriated conservatives and presented an obvious target for reform. In some communities, rabbis tried to limit who could attend. In Mantua, sumptuary laws in 1771 prohibited the host from serving any beverage stronger than coffee, and that only to men engaged in serious study and prayer. With time, the rowdier aspects of precircumcision ceremonies dwindled away, partly in response to regulation and partly as the result of rabbis' emphasis on the sacred meaning of circumcision. Yet in many European communities, these persisted well into the nineteenth century. Subsequently, as Israeli scholar Elliott Horowitz has observed, "the tradition of gaiety and festivity was not entirely lost upon some rabbinical authorities of the twentieth century, who, while recommending prayer and study on the night before the circumcision, nonetheless saw fit to inform their readers that 'in times past it had been customary to dance and to rejoice.'"[48]

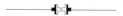

Opposition to circumcision within Judaism may have existed earlier, but the earliest formal objection appears to have arisen in 1843 in Frankfurt. There a party of Jewish laymen founded the Society for the Friends of Reform, a liberal group that published a public manifesto attacking the authority of the Talmud and denying the value of traditional religious ideas and practices. Among the society's breaks with the rabbis, perhaps most controversial was its repudiation of circumcision. *Berit milah*, the reformers declared, was not a *mitzvah*—a rite ordained by God—but an outworn legacy from Israel's earlier phases, an obsolete throwback to primitive religion.[49]

The rabbinic community issued a fusillade of angry responses. Yet unexpectedly, behind the scenes some rabbinic leaders found themselves to be in sympathy with the critics. "I cannot comprehend the necessity of working up a spirit of enthusiasm for the ceremony merely on the ground that it is held in general esteem," privately lamented the eminent scholar, Rabbi Abraham Geiger. "It remains a barbarous bloody act. . . . Its only supports are habit and fear." Like many (though by no means most) of his colleagues, Geiger thought that the idea of blood sacrifice, which had once inspired circumcision, had lost its force, leaving the ritual devoid of substance.[50] For several years, liberal German rabbis struggled with the question of circumcision. Yet the issue was ultimately too divisive, too closely interwoven into the texture of Jewish life and thought, to be debated openly. Jews could declare freedom from the Talmud, one historian has observed, and "they had no trouble dispensing with Hebrew and cutting of their ties to a Jewish Land of Israel." They could even countenance marriage between Jews and Gentiles. "But they could not even consider abrogating circumcision. Moreover, they could not even agree that males who are not circumcised are still Jews!"[51]

European Gentiles may have harbored wild ideas about Jewish ritual practices, but historically few endeavored to outlaw circumcision. Joseph ben David, a German *mohel* operating in France at the end of the eighteenth century, seems to have experienced few legal or social obstacles to plying his trade. Elsewhere, however, there were pockets of resistance. In England, for example, the notorious Jew Bill of 1753 targeted circumcision and *mohels* with special restrictions. One legacy of the Enlightenment, with its confident scientific spirit, was an expanding role for medicine. And as the new medicine, increasingly based on anatomical observation, began to flourish in Paris morgues and German laboratories, certain rationalists cast a cold eye on what they considered a risky and unnecessary surgery on the foreskin. "Tearing with the fingernails does not conform to the principles of rational surgery," declared D. G. M. Salomon, though he allowed that *mohels*, because they were so experienced, probably did a better job with their nails than if they were forced to use scalpels or scissors.[52]

With the emergence of bacteriology, however, the dangers of *periah* seemed trivial compared to *mezizah*. Even before Koch and Pasteur proved the connection between microbes and disease, physicians knew that putting a mouth on an open wound could be a source of contagion. The appearance of hospitals, concentrating doctors and patients in urban centers, made it possible to trace the courses of epidemics. Between 1805 and 1866 at least eight outbreaks of syphilis in various parts of Europe were attributed to infected *mohels*. In 1833, Krakow alone was said to have suffered more than one hundred such cases. At the behest of physicians, various states and municipalities attempted to subject ritual circumcision to some measure of oversight and discipline. In Germany, for example, between 1819 and 1830 a number of regulations followed the pattern of the University of Berlin medical college, requiring not only that ritual circumcisers receive special training in how to resect the foreskin but also that a physician be present to supervise the operation.

Evidence that syphilis and tuberculosis—two of the most feared infectious diseases in the nineteenth century—were spread by *mohels* compelled Jewish physicians to approach their communities' religious leaders. At first they encountered a sense of helplessness. But in the 1840s this changed, largely because an outspoken and famously conservative rabbi in Hungary, Moses Sofer, proclaimed *mezizah* to be dispensable. It had never been an essential part of the covenant, he said, but an invention of cabalists who advanced the notion of *mamtik ha-din* ("mouth and the lips sweeten the Law"). The irony was that *mohels* considered *mezizah* to be a hygienic measure that stopped bleeding and cleansed the wound. In many places, *mohels* who did not suck the wound were thought to have performed an incomplete ritual. Even so, *mezizah* slowly died out in urban centers and communities attuned to modern medical practice.

But elsewhere, in Eastern Europe, in Russia, within islands of orthodoxy in dozens of countries from Germany to the United States, it lingered tenaciously throughout the twentieth century. Sometimes *mohels* used glass or plastic tubes to avoid direct oral-genital contact. Others felt deeply that any compromise of the time-honored practice was a betrayal. In 1994 in New York City, to cite one unsettling episode, the City Department of Health was baffled by the case of a Jewish baby who contracted the HIV virus, even though his mother tested negative. Absent any evidence, the doctors guessed that something mysterious had happened while the baby was in the hospital. They also entertained the possibility, admittedly unlikely, that the virus entered the child's bloodstream during ritual circumcision. When these suspicions surfaced in the press, the incident fueled a growing controversy within the Orthodox Jewish community about the safety of the operation, to child and circumciser alike, in the era of AIDS.

How to deal with the risk of HIV transmission is a matter of sharp disagreement within the rabbinical community. At Yeshiva University, biologist and ethicist Rabbi Moshe Tendler has inveighed against *mezizah b'peh*. "I know from 3,500 years experience that it is safe," he said, "however a mohel who does it now I believe is foolhardy . . . because sadly, the HIV virus has crept into the heterosexual community." In contrast, his colleague, Rabbi

David Bleich, a Talmudic scholar, has maintained that the ritual is in no need of reform. Even *mezizah b'peh* can be rendered safe, he asserted, if the *mohel* first rinses his mouth with 151 proof rum to wipe out any viruses. In practice, he worried that "the danger is more to the circumciser than the baby. . . . The danger to the baby of AIDS is zero unless the mohel has become infected, and I don't know of a single mohel who's become infected." As a precaution, he urged *mohels* to wear gloves and to demand that mothers produce an HIV test before agreeing to operate.[53]

TWO

Christians and Muslims

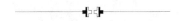

You are circumcised with circumcision, not made by hand in despoiling the body of the flesh, but in the circumcision of Christ, buried with Him in baptism.

—*Colossians 2:11–12*

JESUS, IN KEEPING WITH JEWISH LAW, WAS CIRCUMCISED ON THE EIGHTH DAY (Luke 2:21). But circumcision did not figure into his teachings. Among early Christians, the question of circumcision arose when Jesus' apostles—above all Paul, a Jew steeped in rabbinic tradition—began successfully to proselytize Gentiles. Since the first male followers of Christ were Jews circumcised in infancy, strong voices in the early Church argued that circumcision was compulsory for converts. Yet Paul, a genius of practical evangelism, saw clearly that requiring circumcision would vastly inhibit the appeal of his gospel. In an era of religious ferment, Greek and Roman men might be persuaded to entertain a new theology. Given the ordeal of an operation on the adult penis, though, few would have embraced Christianity if circumcision were a prerequisite.

So, in a brilliant theological stratagem, Paul expanded and reinterpreted the ancient distinction between physical and spiritual circumcision. In his Letter to the Galatians, Paul explained that in the process of instituting a new covenant, a fresh basis for the relationship between God and humankind, Jesus Christ subsumed the old covenant between God and Abraham. Christ, he said, fulfilled the law, and this fulfillment rendered circumcision irrelevant in the eye of God. "In Christ Jesus neither circumcision nor uncircumcision counts for anything," he proclaimed (Galatians 5:6). In Corinth, where a bitter dis-

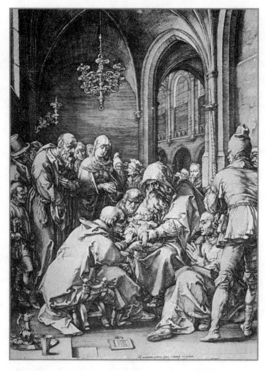

Hendrik Goltzius, *Circumcision of Christ* (1594).

pute broke out when a group of conservative Jewish converts pressured their
Gentile counterparts to become circumcised, Paul was equally adamant: "Was
anyone already circumcised when he was called? Let him not seek to remove
the marks of circumcision. Was anyone uncircumcised when he was called?
Let him not seek circumcision" (1 Corinthians 7:18).

In Pauline theology, faith in Christ eliminated the raison d'être for circumcision: that is, to distinguish Jew from Gentile. Unlike the law of the patriarchs, the new dispensation was to be universal. In his passion to describe a
simple Christian faith that transcended the elaborate, highly codified law he
had grown up with, Paul frequently used circumcision to epitomize the old,
outmoded order. Thus in his tour de force Letter to the Romans he castigated
what he considered Jewish legalism:

> Thou that makest thy boast of the law, through breaking the law dishonourest
> thou God? For the name of God is blasphemed among the Gentiles through
> you, as it is written. For circumcision verily profiteth, if thou keep the law: but
> if thou be a breaker of the law, thy circumcision is made uncircumcision. (Ro-
> mans 2:23–25)

This passage is from the traditional King James Version of the New Testament, which is often euphemistic in regard to sex. In more accurate translation it reads: "If you break the Law, your circumcised glans becomes a foreskin." This was, of course, Paul's central theme: failure to live up to any part of the old covenant made a Jew a sinner, no better than an uncircumcised Gentile. Alternatively, Gentiles who through faith in Christ accepted the "righteousness of the law" would be entitled to be counted as legitimate heirs, equally with Jews, to the covenant of Abraham.

> For he is not a Jew, which is one outwardly; neither is that circumcision, which is outward in the flesh. But he is a Jew, which is one inwardly; and circumcision is that of the heart, in the spirit, and not in the letter; whose praise is not of men, but of God. (Romans 2:28–29)[1]

In view of this argument, what was one to make of God's covenant with Abraham, enshrined, seemingly for all time, by circumcision? Paul insisted that, according to a close reading of the Book of Genesis, "faith was reckoned to Abraham for righteousness" *before* he was circumcised.

> And he received the sign of circumcision, a seal of righteousness of the faith which had yet being uncircumcised: that he might be the father of all them that believe, though they be not circumcised; that righteousness might be imputed unto them also. And the father of circumcision to them who are not of the circumcision only, but who also walk in the steps of that faith of our father Abraham, which he had being yet uncircumcised. For the promise, that he should be the heir of the world, was not to Abraham, or to his seed, through the law, but through the righteousness of faith. (Romans 4:9–13)

This passage proves that the question of circumcision among early Christians was not a peripheral disagreement about preserving or discarding a ritual. It struck to the heart of the new religion, redefining the chosen people.

In Ephesians, an epistle written a generation or so after Paul's death that sought to develop his theological approach more fully, the writer echoes the same theme, reminding his newly converted readers that while they are now heirs to God's promise, they were once "Gentiles in the flesh, those who are called 'foreskin' by those who are called 'circumcision' " (Ephesians 2:11). Aware of the importance of blood shed during *berit milah*, the writer in a fascinating twist suggests that Gentiles, by accepting Christ's blood sacrifice on the cross, are through their faith in him vicariously circumcised.[2]

————————◆▐◆◆▐◆————————

The early Church's cession of circumcision was a crucial aspect of Christianity's transformation from a Jewish sect to a community with a distinct religious identity. Within the communities of early Christianity, believers experienced a powerful sense that Jesus had liberated them from all formal constraints of the law, from circumcision to dietary restrictions. "We Christians eat pork," a Christian speaker boasted in the seventh-century *Trophies of Damascus*, "because He who freed me from circumcision also freed me from abstinence from pork." Nevertheless, Christians accepted the Torah and the other books of the Old Testament literally as the word of God. In consequence, theologians discoursed at length on the question of what, in light of the Gospel of Christ, God had truly intended in the old covenant with Abraham.

Abelard, the twelfth-century French monk and theologian, addressed the problem of circumcision as part of a broader attempt to reconcile the old covenant with the new. In *Dialogue of a Philosopher with a Jew and a Christian*, he held that God had never invented circumcision as a universally binding obligation. Even in the Old Testament, it was not essential to salvation. Enoch, Noah, and Job, not to mention Moses, entered the Kingdom of God without it. Circumcision was, in Abelard's view, a narrow requirement, ordained exclusively for Abraham and his offspring. Since circumcision was not an absolute condition of salvation in the Old Testament and was explicitly rejected by the apostle Paul, the Philosopher in Abelard's dialogue rejects it as obsolete, like the complex temple rituals specified in the Book of Leviticus.[3]

Abelard clarified his argument in two other works, *Commentaries on Romans* and *Sermon on Circumcision*. Once upon a time, he said, the mark had served an essential role. It set Israel apart from the Gentile tribes around them and encouraged Jews to marry within their own group. The appearance of the Messiah, however, dissolved the need for any distinctions. "With the cessation of the Law and the succession of the more perfect Gospels," he wrote, "circumcision has been overtaken by the sacrament of baptism which sanctifies men and women alike." Other theologians expanded on these ideas. Guibert of Nogent, recalling Paul's statement that "in Christ there is neither male nor female," wrote that it was unthinkable that any measure of saving grace would exclude women. Indeed, the *Ysagoge in Theologiam*, providing background on the sacraments, taught that Jesus had replaced circumcision with baptism expressly to include women in the new covenant. Peter Alfonsi, in a similar vein, noted Paul's decree that in Christ, the distinction between Jew and Gentile vanished. Judaism, as Rupert of Deutz explained, was tribal. Mingling with dozens of other desert peoples, the Jews needed a distinguishing characteristic. Christianity's greater destiny, however, was to spread the Gospel to the four corners of the earth; its promise was salvation to all peoples, of all languages and races. Baptism could be applied universally and was, in the teachings of Christ and the apostles, directly linked to salvation. Circumcision, at best, symbolized an outmoded law whose fulfillment had already been realized in Christ.[4]

Not surprisingly, the most rigorous effort to fit circumcision into a grand scheme of Christian theology appeared in the thirteenth century from the Italian quill of St. Thomas Aquinas. In his masterpiece, *Summa Theologica*, the Angelic Doctor systematically introduced objections—for example, "Whether circumcision was instituted in a fitting manner"—that he deflated with point-by-point rebuttals. Here, for instance, is his digression on the relationship between circumcision and sin before Christ's death and resurrection.

> *Objection:* Nothing but sin closes the entrance to the heavenly kingdom. But before the Passion the entrance to the heavenly kingdom was closed to the circumcised. Therefore men were not justified from sin by circumcision.
> *Reply:* Original sin was taken away in circumcision, in regard to the person; but on the part of the entire nature, there remained the obstacle to the entrance of the kingdom of heaven, which obstacle was removed by Christ's Passion. Consequently, before Christ's Passion not even Baptism gave entrance to the kingdom. But were circumcision to avail after Christ's Passion, it would give entrance to the kingdom.[5]

Aquinas concentrated mainly on the spiritual significance of circumcision. Yet others among the Church fathers were interested in something more tangible: they pursued a serious debate about the ontological status of the foreskin of Christ. Faith in the resurrection of the body and images of Christ as a corporeal being sitting at the right hand of God led logically to the question of whether, after the Ascension to heaven he recovered his foreskin. Scholastic theologians eventually realized that this question unfolded into *reductio ad absurdum*. Being flesh and blood, Jesus naturally would have cut his hair, trimmed his nails and lost his umbilical cord. Was the foreskin really all that different from such ordinary detritus? Most churchmen agreed that it was not, though to maintain that the divine foreskin was as trivial as a fingernail seemed dubious in light of the Old Testament record. Nor did the discussion stop there. If a circumcised Christ greeted his uncircumcised followers on Judgment Day, some wondered, would not they be superior to him in physical perfection?

This was unthinkable. In consequence, sages proposed that in order to attain full likeness with Christ, uncircumcised Christians would be divinely circumcised before their entrance into the Kingdom of God.[6]

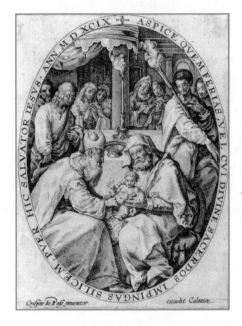

Unlike many of his contemporaries, Dutch artist Crispin de Passe the Elder interpreted the *Circumcision of Christ* (1599) as a formal Jewish ritual. *Charles M. Lea Collection, Philadelphia Museum of Art*

Before and during the Renaissance, throughout Christendom's golden age of relic worship, one of the most prized and most esoteric relics was the foreskin of Christ. One legend held that Mary saved her son's prepuce and carried it about on her person until she ascended to heaven, there to present it to him so that he might stand intact before God the Father. Others, however, suggested that it was left behind and survived. Some people believed that Mary the Mother of Jesus gave it to Mary Magdalene who, before her death, passed it on to the apostles. According to the *Revelations of Saint Birgitta*, a Swedish saint who was canonized toward the end of the fourteenth century, Mary appeared to her in a dream and told how she had preserved the blessed foreskin and finally handed it to Jesus' disciple John. By various means of concealment, the story went, the foreskin survived until the time of Charles the Great in the late eighth century. An angelic courier, in anticipation of Charlemagne's coronation by Pope Leo XIII in the year 800, spirited the relic to him. The emperor, in turn, presented the foreskin to the Church. It remained a private possession of the popes until the sack of Rome in 1527. Purportedly, one of the soldiers of Charles V stole the foreskin, setting the scene for its miraculous recovery. Legend held that the foreskin emitted a sublime odor, much to the delight of grand ladies of Rome. Its rescue and return to Rome was interpreted as a miracle in its own right.[7]

Eroticism was a common undercurrent in medieval and Renaissance treatments of Christ's foreskin. In the mystical vision of the Austrian Agnes Blannbekin (d. 1315), sexual themes are plainly apparent. Agnes was an obscure saint born near Vienna, probably in the mid-thirteenth century. Around the age of eight she began fasting and for the next thirty years refused to eat meat. In her *Via et Revelationes* she described a vision in which she swallowed the divine foreskin. "She feels a small membrane on her tongue, like the membrane of an egg, full of exquisite sweetness." When she touched the membrane with her finger, it slipped down her throat, and "so great was the sweetness at the swallowing of this membrane that she sensed a sweet transmutation through the muscles and organs of her whole body." Afterward, she claimed to have been able to recapture this orgasmic sensation simply by touching her finger to her tongue. St. Anges's transformation of the Eucharist into an erotic fantasy, along with another vision in which she described seeing Jesus nude in a river, struck her clerical superiors as pornographic. Her sainthood notwithstanding, *Via et Revelationes* was long suppressed.[8]

Martin Luther, who wondered how eleven apostles could possibly have twenty-six burial places in Rome alone, marveled at the proliferation of claimants of the holy foreskin. In the sixteenth century, abbeys from Antwerp to Bologna boasted possession of the original vestige. Its healing powers were widely celebrated. In Charroux, the relic was framed in silver and used as a balm for women to alleviate the discomfort of pregnancy and childbirth. A queen of Sicily, diagnosed with an incurable illness, made her pilgrimage to an Italian abbey and claimed that contact with the foreskin of Christ healed her. All the while, dark rumors circulated about nuns abusing these relics, presumably for sexual stimulation.[9]

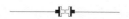

Despite its importance in the Bible, on the eve of the English colonization of North America circumcision was little known in Europe except as an esoteric ritual of Jews and Muslims.

During the late sixteenth and early seventeenth centuries, however, the intellectual winds shifted. In England, a bloody crucible of religious enthusiasm and hostility, we can trace connections between scandalous hearsay about circumcision and long-simmering hostility toward Jews. In 1577 John Foxe, notable for his gruesome *Book of Martyrs*, delivered a *Sermon Preached at the Christening of a Certain Jew, at London*, celebrating the conversion of a Jewish immigrant named Nathaniel Menda. In his opening passages, Foxe railed against the "circumcised Race," denouncing them for their "intolerable Scorpionlike savagenes, so furiously boyling against the innocent infants of the Christian Gentiles: and the rest of your haynous abominations, insatiable butcheries, treasons, frensies, and madnes."[10]

When Foxe insinuated that Jews were fomenting a diabolical conspiracy against Christian babies, he tapped into a dark medieval tradition that had for centuries inspired fear of the Jews. In 1144, a gang of Jews was said to have kidnapped a small boy named William of Norwich, and proceeded to shave his head, torture him, and cut his skin with thorns. Finally, according to chronicler Thomas of Monmouth,

> they lifted him from the ground and fastened him upon the cross. . . . After all these any many and great tortures, they inflicted a frightful wound in his left side, reaching even to his innermost heart. . . . And since many streams of blood were running down from all parts of his body, then, to stop the blood and to wash and close the wounds, they poured boiling water over him.

Explaining the meaning of this episode, Thomas had one of the murderers say, "Even as we condemned the Christ to a shameful death, so let us also condemn the Christian, so that, uniting the Lord and his servant in a like punishment, we may retort upon themselves the pain of that reproach which they impute to us."[11]

More than a century later, in 1255, another Gentile boy of eight or nine, Little Hugh of Lincoln, was found murdered: beaten, nose broken, and circumcised just before his death. This incident sparked a roundup of Jews in the region in which ninety-one were arrested and eighteen executed. During the same period, there was a wave of anti-Semitic practice and regulation. In 1253, for example, royal decrees enforced the 1222 Council of Oxford, which forbade the construction of synagogues, outlawed sexual relations between Jews and Christians, and required Jews to wear identifying badges.[12]

The mystery that shrouded Jewish religious practices—Jews in England and Europe kept their rituals to themselves—ensured that most Protestants remained ignorant and suspicious. On the Continent, in the mid-thirteenth century, as part of a program of Jewish suppression the Catholic Conciliul Viennense, forbade Jews to frequent Christian taverns, dine with Christians, or engage in sexual relations with Christian women. In effect, the council enjoined Christians from converting to Judaism by declaring, "nor may they be circumcised for any reason."[13]

Circumcision was a leitmotif in the stories of Christian boys martyred by Jewish fiends who, in the case of Anderl von Rinn (d. 1462), collected the child's blood in a bowl and used it to make Passover matzohs. The archetypal expression of this atrocity appeared in late fifteenth-century woodcuts illustrating the murder of Saint Simon of Trent. In the wake of a religious uprising shortly before Easter in Trento, Italy, in 1475, the body of a child was discovered near the house of a local Jew. All local Jews were arrested; eight were executed immediately, five later. Simon, meanwhile, was beatified and venerated as a martyr (until 1965, when the Roman Catholic Church withdrew the cult). The prototypal image of Saint Simon's martyrdom, published in Hartmann Schedel's *Nuremberg Chronicle*, portrays Jews circumcising the two-year-old while they bleed him to death, purportedly saving his blood for use in their Passover ritual. Claudine Fabre-Vassas, a French ethnologist, describes a Florentine engraving that depicts the martyrdom:

> The emphasis is placed on the treatment of [St. Simon's] genitals, which are being cut with a large knife. A gaping wound is opened at his throat, from which the blood is flowing into a receptacle. . . . Shearing scissors are ready to cut into his chest and needles pricking his skin contribute to bleeding him white.[14]

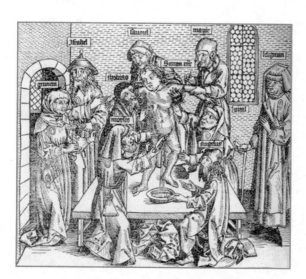

This woodcut of the murder of Simon of Trent clearly depicts his circumcision. *Chronicarum Mundi, Nuremberg, 1493*

This theme was magnified and embellished in seventeenth-century England. "One cruell and (to speak the properest phrase) *Jewish crime* was usuall amongst them," wrote Samuel Purchas, "every yeere towards Easter . . . to steale a young boy, *circumcise him*, and after solemn judgment, making one of their own Nation a Pilate, to crucifie him out of their divellish malice to Christ and Christians."

Was there any basis in fact for Purchas's tale? Certainly there are indications of bizarre practices, as in the *Anglia Judaica* account, "the famous Trial of Jacob of Norwich, and Accomplices, for Stealing away, and Circumcising, a Christian child." In this case, court testimony confirms that a five-year-old boy was abducted while playing in the street and spirited away to Jacob Norwich's house. There his captors blindfolded him and cut off his foreskin. Subsequently, they played a strange game, burying the severed foreskin in a basin filled with dry sand then "blowing the Sand with their Mouths, till they found it again." The winner of the contest declared the boy a Jew. Somehow the boy was returned home and his kidnappers were brought to trial, where his guardians told the court that "by some art or other" the circumcision had been reversed and the boy's foreskin restored.[15]

Unacquainted with circumcision, many people assumed that it amounted to some form of emasculation. Those few Elizabethan Gentiles who did gain admittance to *berit milah* ceremonies and wrote about what they saw were at once fascinated and repulsed. Thomas Coryate, a Londoner who traveled to Constantinople to observe the ritual, left the following chronicle.

[D]ivers Jewes came into the room, and sung certain Hebrew Song; after which the child was brought to his Father, who sate downe in a chaire, and placed the child being now eight days old in his lap. The whole company being desirous that we Christians should observe the ceremonie, called us to approach neere to the child. And when we came, a certaine other Jew drawing forth a little instrument made not unlike those smal Cissers that our Ladies and Gentlewomen doe much use, did with the same cut off the Prepuce of fore-skinne of the child, and after a very strange manner, unused (I believe) of the ancient Hebrews, did put his mouth to the child's yard, and sucked up the bloud. All his Privities (before he came into the roome) were besprinkled with a kind of powder, which after the Circumciser had done his businesse, was blowed away by him, and another powder cast on immediately. After he had dispatched his worke . . . he took a little strong wine that was held in a goblet by a fellow that stood neere him, and powred it into the child's mouth to comfort him in the middest of his paines, who cried out very bitterly; the pain being for the time very bitter indeed, though it will be (as they told me) cured in the space of foure and twentie houres. Those of any riper yeeres that are circumcised (as too often commeth to passe, that Christians that turne Turkes) as at fortie or fiftie years of age doe suffer great paine for the space of a moneth.[16]

Later Europeans would comment on other aspects of Jewish circumcision that struck them as alien or grotesque. Johann Bodenschatz was intrigued by the tradition of posthumous circumcision of infants. If a male baby died before the eighth day, he wrote, his foreskin would be excised, even in the coffin at graveside, so that he would not be buried with that emblem of shame or sin. Just what the Jews did with any foreskin after excision was a question that invited cabalistic speculation. One popular legend held that the Jews buried it in sand in order that a serpent might devour it, thus linking circumcision to snake worship and, more subtly, to the primal myth of rebirth and renewal symbolized by the snake shedding its skin.[17]

Beyond lurid speculation about the mysteries of Jewish ritual, some English churchmen and poets explored the ritual's symbolic meanings in relation to the life of Christ. To the Puritans in the early seventeenth century, every aspect of the Old Testament, every nuance of Mosaic law, constituted foreshadowings and types of Christ. Richard Crashaw (1613–1649), an erudite stylist known for his High Church inclinations, penned an extraordinary poem, "Our Lord in His Circumcision to His Father," in which he imagined the infant Jesus, on the eighth day after his miraculous birth, addressing God the Father.

> *To thee these first fruits of my growing death*
> *(For what else is my life?) lo I bequeath.*
> *Taste this, and as thou lik'st this lesser flood*
> *Expect a Sea, my heart shall make it good.*
> *Thy wrath that wades here now, ere long shall swim*
> *The flood-gate shall be set wide op for him.*
> *Then let him drink, and drink, and do his worst,*
> *To drown the wantonness of his wild thirst.*
> *Now's but the Nonage of my pains, my fears*
> *Are yet but in their hopes, not come to years.*
> *The day of my dark woes is yet but morn.*
> *My tears but tender and my death new-born.*
> *Yet may these unfledg'd griefs give fate some guess,*
> *These Cradle-torments have their towardness.*
> *These purple buds of blooming death may be,*

Erst the full stature of a fatal tree.
And till my riper woes to age are come,
This knife may be the spear's "Praeludium."

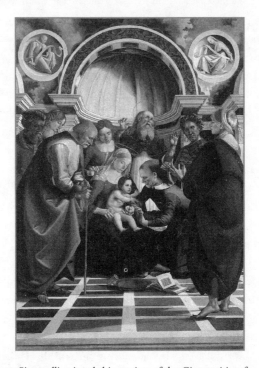

Luca Signorelli painted this version of the Circumcision for
the church of San Francesco around 1491. But the figure of
Jesus was painted over a generation later by Giovanni Antonio
Bazzi (known as Sodoma) in a more sentimental style.
National Gallery, London

The genius here is Crashaw's treatment of the venerable scholastic conceit
that Christ *twice* sacrificed his blood to God the Father, first in the cradle,
then on the cross. Circumcision, with its "lesser flood" of blood, presages
crucifixion, the *mohel*'s blade a precursor of the Roman spear that pierced Jesus' side.[18]

In "Upon the Circumcision," John Milton, the greatest English poet of the
mid-seventeenth century, discovered similar meanings.

He, who with all Heav'n's heraldry whilere
Enter'd the world, now bleeds to give us ease;

Alas, how soon our sin
　Sore doth begin
　　His infancy to seize!

The burden of mankind's sin, which Christ has come to expiate, causes his sufferings to begin in infancy.

And that great Cov'nant which we still transgress
Entirely satisfi'd,
And the full wrath beside
Of vengeful Justice bore for our excess,
And seals obedience first with wounding smart
This day; but Oh! Ere long
Huge pangs and strong
　Will pierce more near his heart.

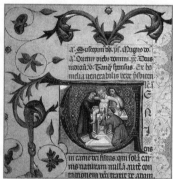

Left: The Circumcision of Christ, from a fourteenth-century French illuminated manuscript. In this depiction, the ritual is not communal but semi-private, conducted by three Jewish men behind closed doors.

Right: Cosimo Tura, *The Circumcision* (ca. 1460). *Isabella Stewart Gardner Museum.*

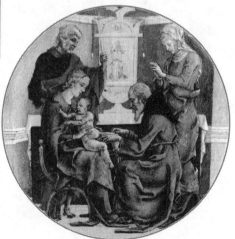

Thus, in Milton's view, Christ's fulfillment of the old covenant—the unforgiving code "which we still transgress"—looks forward to the bloody fulfillment of the new covenant at Golgotha.[19]

————————◀▯▶————————

The dominance of Christianity in Europe meant that Western culture would locate circumcision within a shared historical framework: a Judeo-Christian historical tradition reaching back to Abraham and, ultimately, to the story of creation in the Book of Genesis. But outside Europe and the Mediterranean basin—in the Middle East, Africa, the continent of Australia, and the archipelago of Indonesia and beyond—were other cultures, other traditions that, when became known, would challenge the European worldview.

Above all was Islam. After the fall of the Roman Empire, the tumultuous eastern Mediterranean world was beset by centuries of seething ethnic and sectarian warfare between the Byzantine and Persian empires, and waves of Black Death, famine, and economic disruption. During the sixth century, out of this deeply disordered milieu arose a compelling religious vision of extraordinary power that promised to bring order and meaning to chaos.

The prophet Muhammad (570–632) began life as an indigent orphan, roaming the streets of Mecca. Making his way in the world, he achieved success and wealth as a merchant. Then, at age forty, he experienced a divine calling and a series of visions that revealed to him God's purposes and furnished the content for a new scripture: the Qur'an. In his later years, Muhammad established himself as a prophet in the mold of the biblical patriarchs. His words and deeds became sacred to his followers, and the religious movement that followed exerted phenomenal appeal. By the year Muhammad died, Islam dominated Arabia. In 637 it conquered Iran. Within a century, it had swept through Egypt, Persia, North Africa, then, as traders increased the flow of goods and people, into India, Southeast Asia, Sumatra, and Java and Borneo. Before the Crusades polarized the Mediterranean world, Islam preached kinship and coexistence with Jews and Christians, who, according to the Qur'an, shared the Muslims' heritage as "People of the Book."

There is no reliable evidence that Muhammad himself considered circumcision a vital expression of faith. In the centuries after his death, however, his followers subjected the comparatively simple monotheism of the Prophet to extensive theological elaboration and commentary. In transforming the inspired visions of the Qur'an into practical orthodoxy, Muslim clerics and scholars vigorously debated what the Prophet and his circle said and thought about innumerable matters, large and small. An enduring legacy of this discussion was *hadith*, the sayings of Muhammad, which gradually assumed the authority of revelation, becoming the basis for much Islamic law and practice.

Muhammad, according to some traditions, was born circumcised. (The logic behind this idea is that since circumcision constitutes a superior state of being, the Prophet, in his perfection, must have been distinguished from birth.) Other accounts hold that he was circumcised on the seventh day. In fact the Qur'an is silent about this, as it is about circumcision generally. Nonetheless, Islam has drawn from additional sources of authority, beginning with the Old Testament. Both the Qur'an and the sayings of Muhammad venerate Abraham as "a guide for the people" and a model in all things for the Muslim faithful (Qur'an 2:124; 16:123). Like Moses in the Torah, Muhammad is presented as the latter-day messenger of the religious truth God originally revealed to Abraham. Hence, in the eyes of the faithful, the examples of Abraham and Muhammad have been seen as sufficient reason to circumcise.

Tradition, however, includes several sayings attributed to the Prophet that confirm the ritual's significance. In one of these, Muhammad, addressing a new convert to Islam, commanded him, "Shave off your unbeliever's hair and be circumcised." On another occasion, reacting to the idea that requiring such a painful operation would discourage converts, Muhammad was adamant, "Let him who becomes a Muslim be circumcised, even if he is old." Asked whether an uncircumcised man could go on a pilgrimage, a central feature of Islamic life, Muhammad replied: "Not as long as he is uncircumcised." In the most widely accepted tradition, he is supposed to have taught that "circumcision is a sunnah for men and a makrumah for women." Here the term *sunnah* has been interpreted to mean a practice directly within the tradition of the Prophet himself. It is an obligation tantamount to a commandment. *Makrumah* is weaker, though it suggests that female circumcision is indeed a blessing that would improve a woman. More specifically, Muhammad is reported to have prescribed cutting the foreskin as a *fitrah*, a measure of personal cleanliness that reflects a man's mental and moral health. "Five norms define *fitrah*: circumcision, shaving the pubic hair, moustache trimming, paring the nails, and plucking hair under the armpits." These are supposed to have originated with Allah Himself, who assigned them as refinements on the road to spiritual perfection.[20]

Commentators through the centuries have striven to add theological depth to Muslim circumcision. In a deduction that mirrors rabbinic thinking, the modern Islamist teacher al-Sukkari reasoned that because Allah created circumcision as a type of perfection, Adam, the original perfect man, must have been circumcised at creation.[21] After the Fall, Adam's descendants neglected circumcision, just as they ignored the bulk of God's commandments.

It remained for Abraham to reconfirm the obligation that had existed between God and the first man. A quaint variation on the theme of Adam's circumcision surfaces in one scholar's recital of a Gnostic tradition according to which Adam, in a fit of self-reproach after his original sin, swore that he would cut his own body. The archangel Gabriel overheard him, and in order to save Adam from swearing a false oath, magically gave him a foreskin, which Adam proceeded to cut off. As a result, asserted the sage, Abd-al-Razzaq, "each descendant must fulfil Adam's oath and be circumcised."[22]

In recent times, Muslim leaders have staunchly reaffirmed the religious significance of male circumcision. Some clerics insist that the foreskin traps impurities in the body, causing Allah to turn a deaf ear to the prayers of the unclean. Others point out that if person is found dead among corpses on a battlefield, only if he is circumcised he will be prayed for and properly buried in a Muslim cemetery. At the extreme, the Shafite school of Islamic law, which is predominant in eastern Africa and Indonesia, has taken the position that Muslim men may be forced to submit to the procedure. The Ibadites maintain that marriage to an uncircumcised Muslim is null and void, whether or not the marriage has been consummated. Al-Sukkari has written in defense of a woman's right to revoke her marriage to an uncircumcised man because the foreskin is repulsive and potentially a source of contagion. Others have argued for extensions of Islamic family law that would deny an uncircumcised man the rights of guardianship or to give his consent to the marriage of a female relative. Within the world of Islam, the consensus is overwhelming that an uncut man is a second-class citizen.

Thus, for most Muslims, circumcision is automatic. Unlike Jewish *berit milah*, however, it has never been standardized into common ritual. Whereas Jewish law places great emphasis on the eighth day after birth, Muslim clerics have never agreed on the best time for the operation. Some, supposing that Muhammad himself was circumcised on the seventh day, have insisted that this is the ideal time for the operation; others abhor the suggestion of imitating a Jewish practice. Muslim sage Wahb ibn Munabbih, questioned about whether or not to circumcise on the seventh day, advocated doing so "to make it easy for the child." British anthropologist Robertson Smith's 1927 observation still holds true: "Circumcision, which was originally a preliminary to marriage, and so a ceremony of introduction to the full prerogative of manhood, is now generally undergone by Mohammedan boys before they reach maturity."[23] British and American neonatal circumcision, done for medical reasons shortly after birth, influenced some Muslims, particularly the better educated and those living in urban centers, to operate in infancy. If there is any consensus, it is that the surgery is better done in infancy or early childhood than later, when youths become less compliant. Should a child grow to puberty without being cut, however, circumcision becomes mandatory before he can participate in the actions of worship. Ibnul-Qayyim declared: "It is obligatory upon the guardian to circumcise the child so that he attains puberty and has been circumcised—since this is something essential for the accomplishment of an obligation."

Muslim religious leaders have made efforts to vindicate circumcision on medical grounds. At the First International Conference for the Scientific Aspects of Qur'an and Sunnah, held in Islamabad, Pakistan, in 1987, Islamic scholars reviewed a series of studies published in American medical journals in which physicians sought to prove that the procedure remained a prudent preventive measure against diseases like urinary tract infection and penile cancer. "The performance of circumcision and the practice of Sunan Al-Fitra as recommended in Islam is medically beneficial," the panel concluded, "and reflects the wisdom of the Islamic statements."[24]

As for the cutting itself, the Islamic scholar al-Mawardi declared, "The ideal method is to remove the skin completely from the beginning of the glans, and the minimum condition is that nothing is left to cover the end of the glans." In most cases, the Muslim operation has been more conservative than its Jewish counterpart, for there is no history of circumcision reversal in Islam, hence no need for *periah*, the radical ablation of the foreskin. Ritual circumcisers never achieved in Islam the status that *mohels* attained in Judaism. The multitude of tribal religions and sacramental practices subsumed by Islam has meant that the operation, the person who performs it, and the ceremony surrounding circumcision vary dramatically from place to place. In the early twentieth century, for instance, an ethnographer surveying Turkey and Arabia found that most procedures were performed by barbers using razors. "Tying up the foreskin with two threads," he wrote, "it is also simply drawn out and severed with a diagonal cut." To aid healing, some circumcisers dipped the cut penis into a fresh egg white mixture, then wrapped it in oilcloth. Others treated the wound with dirt, sand, wax, animal fat, or mud. In many communities, after the operation was finished and the child had returned home to recuperate, members of his family would spread cumin seeds on his bed to thwart spirits that might hinder healing.

In a circumcision ceremony in the African Republic of Mali, one writer found Muslim youths alongside boys from unconverted families, each waiting his turn for an operation performed by the village blacksmith. Malinke convention required the boy to stand stoically, facing east, a circumcised relative standing behind him. (The adult's job was to catch the boy if he fainted or, in rare instances, to hold him if he struggled or tried to flee.) Working swiftly, the blacksmith seized the boy's penis with the fingers of his left hand. He stretched the prepuce beyond the end of the glans, then he used his fingernail to make a line in the skin, tracing where to cut. He cut the extended foreskin almost even with the tip of the glans; when it retracted, the glans was left exposed. The resulting wound was washed with ointment made of local saba fruit, then dressed with sana leaves and tied with string. After three days, the leaf bandage was removed. Until it healed completely, the wound was treated with peanut soap and water and a paste of local herbs.[25]

In recent decades, as Islam has been swept by waves of fundamentalism and dreams of religious purity, circumcision has served as a unifying symbol and often as a token of religious conquest. Remarking on the vigor of Islam's religious imperialism, V. S. Naipaul writes, "There probably has been no imperialism like that of Islam and the Arabs. The Gauls, after 500 years of Roman rule, could recover their old gods and reverences; those beliefs hadn't died; they lay just below the Roman surface. But Islam seeks as an article of faith to erase the past; the believers in the end honor Arabia alone; they have nothing to return to." Circumcision is a vital symbol of this religious imperialism, which unites disparate peoples by gradually subsuming their sacred past into a kind of Islamic folk religion. In Islam proper, circumcision is predominantly a personal rite, a measure of individual purification. An indelible sign, in imitation of the Prophet, it commits a man permanently to his faith.[26]

Yet this fundamental conceit is only the common thread linking dozens, perhaps hundreds, of different circumcision rituals conducted under the banner of Islam. Anthropologist Ruth Benedict once remarked of rituals that "the instability of the associated symbolic meaning is as striking as the stability of seemingly arbitrary ritual acts." Circumcision is perhaps typical insofar as the physical act of cutting continues but with changing significance.

As carried out in Indonesia, Africa, and elsewhere circumcision is intensely communal. And communal meanings, with ancient roots into tribal pasts, differ as markedly as the histories and totemic memories they evoke. The ritual is so deeply embedded that its power is mostly taken for granted. Perhaps this is because it smoothly connects what converts to Islam understand to be the progressive force of their religion with the primeval customs of their native lands. Many converted peoples look back to aboriginal animist traditions that include genital cutting. By allowing these traditions to flow freely into its reservoir, Islam in effect modernizes them, and enables them to connect with a sacred global order.[27]

One window into a single set of tribal meanings of circumcision appears in a field study conducted during the early 1960s by a young British anthropologist named Emanuel Marx. Living for a year and a half among four Negev Bedouin tribes, who farmed the Beersheba Plain in southern Israel (a region Abraham is said once to have occupied), Marx had a chance to study their circumcision rituals at first hand. For the Negev, the circumcision of a son offered the tribes' wealthiest members an occasion to stage an elaborate feast. These feasts, lasting from ten days to two weeks before the operation and costing "an amount equal to an average Bedouin family's annual income," eclipsed the circumcision itself. The host set up a special "feast-camp," and to this camp traveled groups of visitors from around the region. Depending on the tribal customs of the sponsor, the affair either featured lively celebrations and sports such as horse and camel racing, or else proceeded in "dignified silence." But in all cases the feast-giver, by sponsoring the event, demonstrated his superior status. Poorer fathers, unable to afford feasts of their own, took advantage of the larger event to have their own boys circumcised. Throughout the long ceremony, these men served in a subordinate role as helpers.[28]

After many days of eating, singing, gift giving, social and business conversation in which people who rarely saw each other renewed important relationships, the actual circumcision was anticlimactic. At the appointed time, women filed out of their guest-tent, where the cutting was to take place, chanting "Oh circumciser, be your hand light" (a plea to make the surgery as painless as possible). When they finished and dispersed, the operator entered the tent. Meanwhile, adult men fanned out through the camp to round up the boys who were to be cut. Marx was told that the boys had fled in panic, but he saw "no signs of fear in them. They had good appetites and played around the camp." Indeed, until that moment nobody had paid much attention to them, "for the feast had been arranged chiefly in order to demonstrate the wealth of the feast-giver and to renew gift-links. The circumcision seemed to provide an acceptable pretext for feasting."[29]

Boys entered the tent accompanied by a paternal uncle or another older male; the boys' fathers and mothers remained on the sidelines. The circumciser operated on the boys as they sat on the knees of the man who held them. Although the operator was known to be a devout man, the event itself was devoid of religious embellishment. With no prayer, no sacred song or verse, the circumciser simply set about his work "to the accompaniment of music from a transistor radio." When he finished, the boys were handed over to their parents. For consolation, they were given sweets to eat but otherwise received no special treatment. In minimizing the religious significance of the act to almost nothing, the Bedouin revealed an extreme attitude, and one that is reflected in their language. According to one scholar, they do not use the ordinary Arab term for circumcision (*tuhûr*, literally, "cleansing"), but speak simply of "cutting the boys." Underscoring the secular character of the Bedouin operation, Marx discovered that in one of the feasts he attended the surgeon was a *mohel*, a Jew from Beersheba hired for his technical prowess, and that no Muslim had even been considered for the task.[30]

These Bedouin were exceptional; in other places language evokes profound connections between the ritual and the religious community. In Java, circumcision is translated as "welcoming a boy into the bosom of Islam." In the former French colonial city of Algiers, where religious practice mixes elements of Catholicism and Islam with local animist beliefs, villagers expect to receive printed invitations from friends and relatives to attend a baby boy's "bapt^me" or baptism, that is, his circumcision.[31] Slowly, under pressure from Islam, throughout the world the traditional structures of the old rite are transformed. In rural African villages, the circumcising witch doctor gives way to the Muslim cleric. In the mountains of Indonesia, where some children were circumcised soon after birth and others wait until adolescence, the cutting once performed at a feast by the community's ritual circumciser, the local *dukon sonnat*, is now done on a stainless steel table by a paramedic.[32]

An excellent illustration of the fusion of primitive mysticism and modern Islamic motifs is the circumcision ceremony in the Javanese Sultanate of Yogyakarta. There, with the possible exception of marriage, circumcision is the defining event in a young man's coming of age. It signifies his entry into the *umat*, the Islamic community of faith. The feasts surrounding circumcision blend entrance into Islam with affirmations of Javanese social hierarchy. American anthropologist Mark Woodward has captured some of the facets of this transition in his description of a *slametan*, a ritual meal honoring the circumcision of the grandson of a Yogyakarta prince.

> The boy was eleven when his grandfather decided that he was old enough to be circumcised. On the day of the ceremony, he was taken in a small motorcade to the clinic owned by a famous *tukang supit* [holy man specializing in circumcision] approximately thirty miles from Yogyakarta. . . . He looked very much like a young boy dressed for the Friday service at the mosque (normally he wore Western clothing).

When he appeared at the feast held in his honor later the same evening, the boy's aspect was utterly different.

He wore the complete Javanese ceremonial costume consisting of a batik *kain* (a long skirt made from a single piece of material that is wrapped around the body in a complicated way), a silk waistcoat similar to that worn by a *pangerani* (prince), a jeweled brooch, a turban, and, most important a *keri*. He looked, and was treated, like a young prince.

Curious about this striking metamorphosis, Woodward queried the boy's grandfather. By being circumcised, the old man explained, his grandson had become a man and was henceforth expected to comport himself as one. As part of initiating his grandson into the company of men, circumcision entitled the young man to wear the *keri*, heirlooms thought to possess magical powers so potent that children are forbidden to handle them.[33]

Circumcision is so ingrained in Islamic life that opposition has been almost inconceivable. For those tempted to raise doubts, the theocratic impulse—most aggressive in countries like Iran and Afghanistan, but present in most Muslim communities—has struck swiftly to quash dissent on matters of *sunnah*.

In recent years, questioning circumcision in any respect has been assailed by militant Islamists as blasphemy. For instance, when a retired Libyan judge, Mustafa Kamal al-Mahdawi, published a book that questioned the legitimacy of the ritual, he came under furious attacks from the clergy and the press. Basically, al-Mahdawi argued that as a Jewish custom, originating in ancient superstitions of the Israelites, circumcision deserved no standing in Islam. In

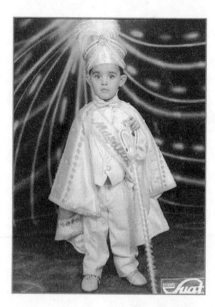

A Turkish boy from a wealthy family dressed in his circumcision suit.

response, in the summer of 1992, the preacher of the Mosque of the Prophet in Medina, Saudi Arabia, hastily issued a tract that was printed in bulk, flown to Libya and widely distributed. In it he urged the Muslim Arab League and the Islamic Conference to organize a fatwa of all Muslim scholars against al-Mahdawi unless he retracted his apostasy. Meanwhile, his book was removed from shops and libraries, and burned. At bottom, the judge's offense was to deny "that male circumcision is compulsory when there is unanimity in favour of it and when Mohammed was Himself circumcised." In the wake of the Salman Rushdie affair, al-Mahdawi was hardly disposed to make light of the death threat hanging over him.[34]

THREE

Symbolic Wounds

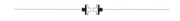

The mutilation of the genitals among the various savage tribes of the world presents a strange and unaccountable practice of human ideas, which one is not able to reconcile with any reasoning power. Why such customs should be in vogue none can tell at the present time; but we must suppose that at some period they had their significance, which in the course of ages has been lost, and the practice has been handed down from generation to generation.

— *J. Henry C. Simes, "Circumcision" (1890)*

THE LATE FIFTEENTH CENTURY SAW THE DAWNING OF THE AGE OF DISCOVERY, a time when European adventurers circumnavigated the globe, exploring the coasts and rivers of Africa, pushing deep into the Americas, and confronting exotic cultures no European had ever seen. Ships returning from their years at sea brought strange reports from explorers, traders, missionaries, and later, colonial administrators. Inexplicably, it came to light that tribes in remote parts of the world—Africa, the Americas, Australia, and Indonesia—performed a bewildering variety of circumcisionlike surgeries on both males and females. In males, these operations ranged from nicking or trimming off just the tip of the foreskin to a disfiguring mutilation that involved cutting the underside of the penis through the urethra all the way from the meatus to the scrotum.

What could explain these far-flung rituals? European travelers' first impulse was to assume that primitive folk in strange lands must have shared a common ancestry with the Jews. If the origins of humankind, as the Bible taught, traced from Adam through Noah and his sons, perhaps remote tribes had inherited circumcision from some anciently dispersed patriarch. Speculating about the fate of the so-called lost tribes of Israel, Londoner Thomas Thorowgood, in a book called *Jews in America* (1660), decided that "many Indian Nations are of Judaicall race, seeing this frequent and constant Character of Circumcision, so singularlie fixed to the Jews, is to be found among them." By the end of the eighteenth century, however, as the European literature of tribal observation mushroomed, trying to link every circumcising tribe back to ancient Israel came to seem absurd.[1]

Questions nonetheless remained: If the heathen had not inherited it from Israel, where did circumcision come from? If tribal cutting was not a corrupt version of God's covenant with Abraham, what did it mean? The first matter, which prompted endless guesswork and speculation, remains unanswerable. The second question—about ritual meaning—called for the disciplines we now think of as cultural anthropology or ethnography.

In the middle part of the nineteenth century, a handful of scholars (mainly British explorers) began to develop increasingly formal techniques of cultural investigation. Of these, Sir Richard Burton is probably the best known. Burton was captivated by the folkways and rituals of exotic cultures, especially any practices and beliefs related to sex. In 1853 he had himself circumcised in order to pass for a Muslim and avoid exposure when he traveled to the forbidden city of Mecca. Burton wrote forty-three volumes describing his explorations among tribal peoples in India, Africa, and the Americas. Meanwhile, in a few European academic centers, techniques and a body of knowledge slowly emerged that were analytic, relying on observation and description to locate certain behaviors (such as initiation rituals, which would become a primary focus) within larger patterns of social meaning. The subsequent work of nineteenth-century scholars such as Andrew Lang and James G. Frazer (though they relied mainly on secondhand observations) introduced both functional interpretation and comparative analysis in dissecting rituals, gauging their prevalence and elaborateness and extracting common themes and motifs from culture to culture. They loved classification and taxonomic schemes capable of "organizing" the chaotic variations of tribal practice.[2]

American anthropologist Lewis Henry Morgan wrote in *Ancient Society* in 1877, "It is undeniable that portions of the human family have existed in a state of savagery, other portions in a state of barbarism, and still other portions in a state of civilization. . . . It seems equally so that these three distinct conditions are connected with each other in a natural as well as necessary sequence of progress." Indeed, beginning as early as the 1840s (nearly two decades before the publication of Charles Darwin's *Origin of Species*), the organizing principle for cultural analysis was evolution. James Frazer, author of the tremendously influential work *The Golden Bough*, described an evolutionary sequence in which simple, primitive peoples exemplified the early phases of social development through which modern societies were thought to have passed long ago. Frazer's magnum opus, like Ernest Crawley's *Mystic Rose* (1902), compiled an immense stock of stories and observations of varying reliability taken from missionaries, traders, and adventurers. In Frazer's scheme, isolated tribes like the Australian aborigines merited close attention chiefly for what they could reveal about the early phases of modern man's development. Such living fossils, to his way of thinking, made it possible to peer almost directly into the past.

According to Frazer's progressive model, humankind passed through three stages: magic, religion, and science. Within this scheme, religious circumcision as practiced by the Jews contained ancient magical elements, like sucking the bloody wound, that linked it to the world's most archaic rites. Frazer considered initiation to be "the central mystery of primitive society," an expression of societies' desperate drive to control sex and death. Thus, in his view, the initiation rite of circumcision was essentially sacrificial. One small part of a tribe member's body (his foreskin) was sacrificed to the divine powers to redeem the community.[3]

Succeeding generations of scholars proposed different interpretations. Generally, though, they tended to share Frazer's progressive view of history and his evolutionary assumptions about cultural development. Among the cleverest and best known was Mircea Eliade, a scholar at the University of Chicago whose *Rites and Symbols of Initiation* (1958) attracted a large following among anthropologists and historians of religion. Eliade described the rituals of the Australian aborigines as crude expressions of ideas—sacrifice, life after death, and so forth—that would realize their ultimate historical refinement in Christianity. Studying "primitives," his real interest was to track down the origins of modern beliefs. Eliade explained the spiritual development of humanity in terms of global advancement, a ladder of increasingly refined religious thought and ritual practice on which each society occupied a distinct rung.

An imaginative writer, Eliade moved smoothly between acute observation and implausible conjecture. He noticed, for example, that certain African tribes cloaked ritual circumcisers in symbolism (masks, leopard skin capes, inscribed staffs) associated with wild beasts. What this signified, he concluded, was that "the masters of initiation are divinities in animal form, which supports the hypothesis that structurally the ritual belongs to an archaic hunter culture."[4] No matter which cultures practiced it, ritual circumcision was to be construed as an expression of ancient beliefs. The job of the anthropologist was to unearth those core beliefs, ideally in their most primitive forms, and then to reveal how certain archetypal ideas reemerged time after time in specific rites in different cultures.

Many years earlier the French social theorist Émile Durkheim had developed an opposite approach, and one that would prove far more illuminating. From his post at the University of Paris, Durkheim pursued a functional sociology, a method that balanced robust empiricism with rigorous theory. The trouble with Frazer's approach and those who follow it, he wrote, is that it assumed that ideas existed independently from the individual rituals that conveyed them. This was a form of Platonism that failed to explain how ideas—particularly the kind of shared ideas expressed in religious rituals—actually took shape within the social order.

With respect to circumcision, the earliest proponent of a functional, sociological methodology was a young Belgian scholar, Arnold van Gennep. Three years before Durkheim published his watershed treatise on Australian totemic systems, *Les Formes Elémentaires de la vie religieuse* (1912), van Gennep produced a brilliant behavioral analysis of initiation rituals, *Les Rites de passage* (1909).

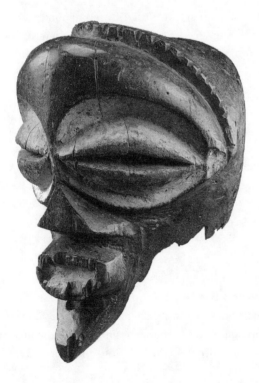

The dramatic Kalelwa mask, used by the Jokwe in Angola. According to Marie-Louise Bastin, an anthropologist at the University of Brussels, Jokwe boys were circumcised during an extended ordeal in the bush, where masked tribesmen donned a variety of masks to evoke different aspects of the cosmos.

Like Durkheim, he was an empiricist and insisted that the primary task of anthropology was to examine human behavior—particularly behavior that societies invested with exceptional meaning, like rituals and ceremonies—in the full social setting in which they operated. Simply put, one could not hope to understand a ritual without analyzing all of the behavior and symbolism associated with it. Describing the ways circumcision functioned within various tribal groups, van Gennep defined it as a pivotal rite of passage, a life-crisis event that signified transition from one social station to another. In every instance van Gennep could find, circumcision manifestly linked physical modification—cutting the penis (or, in females, the external genitalia)—with a change in the initiated person's social position. Though dated, his attempt to gain general intellectual control over the diverse circumcision practices of tribal societies illustrates the complexity of the problem anthropologists faced.[5]

The first thing that puzzled van Gennep was the wide variations in age that different societies chose as the proper time to circumcise. Many tribes along the coast of East Africa, for example, waited until a boy was a few years old. But in Australia and parts of Indonesia, it was common for some communities to time the procedure to coincide roughly with puberty, while others picked earlier ages, seemingly at random. In an extreme case, the Gisu of Uganda were known to cut men well past puberty. Even within small areas—one section of Morocco, for instance—age variation ran from seven or eight days to twelve or thirteen years. Assembling the evidence, van Gennep reckoned that "the same rite sometimes marks the beginning of childhood, sometimes of adolescence, but it has nothing to do with physical puberty." Circumcision was not meant to signify a person's transition from presexual to sexual status. Rather, like a whole array of bodily transformations—ritual haircutting, knocking out teeth, amputating part of the little finger, tattooing, scarring, perforating and stretching the earlobes, the septum, or the lips—the mark of circumcision symbolized the individual's detachment from the mass of humanity and his permanent inclusion in a distinct tribal community.[6]

Van Gennep and others pointed out that male and female circumcision each sought the refinement of the sex organs by excising those parts—prepuce, clitoris, labia—that bore some resemblance to the opposite sex. With the glans permanently exposed, the penis gives the impression of a permanent erection (which is why the ancient Greeks considered circumcision indecent). In the most basic sense, it may look more masculine. Alternatively, communities that practice female genital cutting often say that an uncircumcised woman, because her genitalia protrude (and thus resemble a miniature penis) is not entirely feminine. Taking this notion to the extreme, some East African tribes consider an uncut woman incapable of conception, or, should she conceive, of bearing a healthy baby.[7]

The broad explanatory scheme van Gennep advanced deeply influenced his peers and successors, especially as it came to apply to coming-of-age rituals. It is succinctly described in a passage from anthropologist Bronislaw Malinowski.

> The novices have to undergo a more or less protracted period of seclusion and preparation. Then comes initiation proper, in which the youth, passing through a series of ordeals, is finally submitted to an act of bodily mutilation: at the mildest, a slight incision or the knocking out of a tooth; or, more severe, circumcision; or, really cruel and dangerous, an operation such as subincision. . . . The ordeal is usually associated with the idea of death and rebirth of the initiated one, which is sometimes enacted in a mimetic performance. But besides the ordeal, less conspicuous and dramatic, but in reality more important, is the second main aspect of initiation: the systematic instruction of the youth in sacred myth and tradition, the gradual unveiling of tribal mysteries and the exhibition of sacred objects.

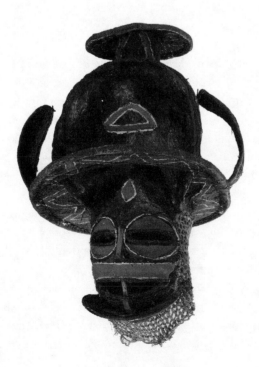

Mbagani circumcision mask from Zaire, probably dating from the late nineteenth century.

This statement accurately applies to societies that practice rites of initiation. Yet it does not address the question of why such rites are present in one society yet absent in another.[8]

Since overarching interpretations have tended to break down under analysis, losing persuasive power whenever scholars have tried to reconcile practices across different periods and cultures, anthropologists have in recent years tended to lower their sights, settling for thick description of the symbolic and functional aspects of circumcision.

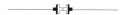

In the history of nineteenth- and twentieth-century anthropology, no tribal people attracted more attention for their various genital mutilations than the aboriginal folk of Australia. When Dutch explorers first set foot on Australian soil early in the seventeenth century, as many as 700 tribes lived on the continent, their origins stretching back perhaps 60,000 years. After European settlement began in earnest in 1788, colonization steadily took its toll, reducing the native population through disease and relentless economic oppression. With the emergence of anthropology in the late nineteenth century, however, the Aborigines came to be prized as a unique human resource. The fascination of studying these tribes lay in the idea that Australia, owing to its isolation from modernizing and cross-cultural influences, offered scholars a time warp where they could study, as the pioneering anthropologist Baldwin Spencer put it, "human beings that still remain on the culture level of men of the Stone Age."[9]

Spencer, along with F. J. Gillen, trekked deep into the Outback in the 1890s. For the next thirty years they studied dozens of aboriginal tribes, particularly the Arunta. Their accounts, and those of Herbert Basedow, a German-trained physician and anthropologist of the pith helmet school who served as Australia's Chief Medical Inspector and Protector of Aborigines in the Northwest Territory during the 1920s, constitute an extraordinary source of historical information about rites of passage and genital cutting as they existed in the world's most famous "primitive" culture.[10]

Not that there was a consistent pattern; rites varied greatly within regions and among tribes. Communities that did circumcise (or practice subincision) impressed Europeans with the pageantry surrounding the operation, often elaborately prolonged and gory to the point of being Wagnerian. While there was no such thing as a typical ceremony, many accounts include common elements, making it possible to create a composite portrait.

Not all tribes circumcise, but among those who do, the ritual is public and charged with great significance. Weeks in advance, the approaching event becomes a central preoccupation within the community for everyone, young and old. Deciding when a boy has reached the right age—normally about twelve years—is left to the male members of his family. Instead of sharing their decision with him, however, the boy's brothers, or other older males who act as "designated brothers," catch him unawares and spirit him away to a small outpost they have prepared some distance from the tribe's main encampment. There he remains, confined and closely guarded to prevent contact with other people, especially girls and women.

Typically the area where the ritual will take place is declared off limits to women. The men who will enact the ensuing drama proceed to decorate their bodies garishly with red and white down. Others clear a space in the underbrush, loosen the dirt with sharp sticks, and strew the earth with leaves from a red gum tree. Once these preparations are complete, as the boy looks on, a huge bonfire is ignited. Dancers gather around him, circling the fire, singing, chanting, doing their best to terrify the victim by making ferocious faces. As

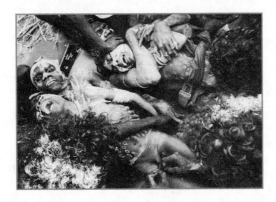

This image of an Australian aboriginal circumcision captures the frenetic intensity of the ritual at the moment of cutting.

the scene builds in intensity, the boy is escorted to a second, smaller fire some distance away. There men smear his body from head to foot with red ochre, truss his hair, then lead him back to the main site.

At this point, with the boy disoriented and mortified, elders approach him to whisper their deepest tribal secrets. (These secrets might include, for example, the locations of holy places and totemic objects.) On pain of death for him and his family, they warn him never to reveal what he has learned. In some tribes, this phase of the ritual consumes days, and includes the blindfolding and unblindfolding of the boy and instruction in performing certain totemic ceremonies.[11]

As the time for the cutting approaches, dancers crowd around the boy, seize him, lift him up and carry him forward. Shrieking and chanting become frenetic, more hands grab at the frightened boy until, suddenly, he is flung down onto the prone bodies of men who have arranged their bodies to form a "human operating table." Lying on their backs, these men pinion the victim, holding his arms and legs, while another man sits on his chest. Aghast at the

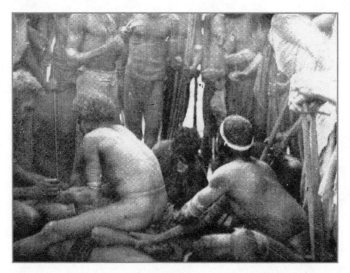

Circumcision of a Wogait boy in Australia. "With his left hand the surgeon seizes the prepuce, whilst a veritable reverberation of short-sounded 'I, I's' meets him from the mouths of all present, and as he draws it well forward a number of hacks severs it." Herbert Basedow, *The Australian Aboriginal* (1925).

violence of the struggle, the onlookers shudder with fear. Men who have undergone initiation themselves dash about vehemently, brandishing burning sticks and shouting into the night.

To prevent his crying out, someone stuffs a hair-string gag into the victim's mouth. The men holding his legs spread them and pull them downward, exposing his pubic area. In an instant, the crowd parts and the ritual circumciser strides toward the boy. He has the aspect of a man entranced, "his beard between his lips and his eyes rolling in their sockets." His hand carries a knife chipped from flint or quartz. Without hesitation he begins the cutting, finally, after several strokes, severing the prepuce. When the operation is finished, the surgeon holds the foreskin aloft to raucous approval. Men prop up the boy, who is bewildered and, in many cases, in shock, allowing his blood to spill onto a piece of bark. The wound is important, and tribes differ in the way they treat it. Some northern tribes, for example, dress it with thin sheets of bark, earth, emu fat, and hot ashes to stop the bleeding. Once the boy regains his senses, he may be presented with a spear or a shield, badges of manhood among the tribe's hunters. While he recovers, the boy stays in the bush apart from the tribe, eating a special diet, closely watched for signs of sickness. At last

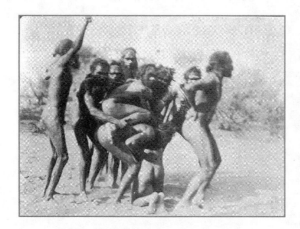

Circumcision ceremony, Kukata tribe in Australia. "Beyond themselves with excitement, they lay hands upon the lad and lift him upon the back of two or three of the men who are stooping in readiness to receive him." Herbert Basedow, *The Australian Aboriginal* (1925).

he returns to the group, wearing a fur tassel over his penis. When they first see him, his mother, sisters, and aunts wail, tearing their hair and pricking their bodies in sympathy for the suffering he has endured.

The psychological and physical harshness of aboriginal procedures is so daunting that when they sense their time approaching, some boys run away, desperately seeking refuge with anyone who will hide them. This is often a sympathetic European. Nevertheless, according to Basedow's account, eventually most fugitives are captured and dragged back home. As punishment and to set an example tribal elders impose an especially excruciating tribulation. "The [fore]skin is stretched forward under considerable tension and severed with a stone knife," he wrote. "In several specimens which are in my possession, the external sheath was cut so high up that a number of pubic hairs were removed with it."[12]

There is no way of telling how long native Australians have practiced circumcision, just as there is no way of knowing its origins. Anthropologist Ashley-Montagu reports that one South Australian tribe attributes the procedure to a mythological feathered creature called *Jurijurilja*. Legend holds that the primordial beast hurled a boomerang that flew back, flaying the foreskin of his penis and, in the same motion, passing through the genitals of his wives. Circumcision and menstrual bleeding are thus explained in a single fable.[13]

"Years ago, when I first learned of subincision—the remarkable practice of cutting the ventral portion of the penile urethra, sometimes from the glans to the scrotum—I puzzled over its meaning," he wrote, "until I found that, among the Errand of Central Australia, the subincized penis was called by the same name as the female vulva." Subincision was intended to reshape the penis in the image of the vulva. The subsequent hemorrhage was likened to menstruation which enabled females naturally to dispose of the evil humors accumulating in their bodies. "To continue the same effect, males periodically engaged in incision of the penis and called it menstruation."[14]

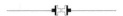

Perhaps the most meticulous attempt to analyze a circumcision ritual in its fuller historical, social, and cultural context and to extract its symbolism is Maurice Bloch's fifteen-year study during the 1960s and 1970s of the Merina of Madagascar.

The Merina circumcise fairly early in life, usually between the ages of one and two years. To them, the idea that a boy would not be circumcised is simply "inconceivable," though when Bloch pressed villagers to explain why they felt so strongly, they were hard put to articulate a reason. Beyond acknowledging the authority of tradition ("Our ancestors have always done this, so we must do it too"), some people spoke of the ritual's making boys "sweet" or "beautiful" and clean. Others added that without circumcision, boys could not become men and might never achieve sexual potency. The most deep-seated belief was simply that circumcision constituted a blessing. In Merina culture, blessing is a concept rich with implication, encompassing the important elements of a child's destiny and his importance to his kin and the larger community.[15]

As with the Bedouins, the event itself has become a defining moment not merely for the child but also for his extended kinship network. Elaborately staged and lavishly expensive, the ceremony is arranged to take place in a cool time of year, because cold weather is thought to make the operation safer. Preparations take place "in an atmosphere of growing excitement and revelry, heightened by the promises of the smell of roasting coffee, the taste of rich food, the intoxication of rum and the exhilaration and tension of familial reunion."

The points of convergence for the ritual are two special houses. One hides the ritual circumciser, an expert hired for the job who must be kept out of view until the moment of the operation. The other is the place where the circumcision will be performed, customarily the boy's parents' home. Their dwelling is transformed into a ritual pagoda. Conforming to precise protocols, a local astrologer supplies medicinal herbs—wild grasses and reeds (sometimes dipped in cattle dung), which are brought into the house along with bananas, sugarcane, and a special gourd, dried and prepared in advance by the initiate's parents. The gourd is a token of communal unity.

The cast of actors is large. First, there is the circumciser who, despite being unrelated, is dubbed "father of the child." In some instances he is an astrologer, supervising the collection of plants, and perhaps selecting the most auspicious day for the event. Then there are "mothers of the child," a group of young unmarried women assigned to dance with him and comfort him through his distress. These "mothers" are enjoined from sexual intercourse any time during the ceremony. Finally, another group, the "youths whose father and mother are still living," serve as intermediaries between the coming generation of the child and the declining generation of his parents. They carry out many tasks essential to the ceremony, such as hauling water and staking and slaughtering a bull in connection with the ceremony.

At the appointed hour, a crowd gathers in front of the circumcision house. A sacrificial bull is tethered to a post. Near the bull, men have laid a mat on the ground, tacked down by a wooden peg in its northeast corner, known as "the corner of the ancestors." The peg signifies contact between the community, the young male about to be cut, and the invisible procession of dead forebears. A bowl of water is placed on the mat, the water covering several uncut silver coins, symbols of holiness and purity. Elders—two male and one female—representing both sides of the boy's family address the assembly, giving an invocation. They call on the power of God and the power of their ancestors.

At length, after repeated invocations, the boys to be circumcised appear, dressed in white smocks and accompanied by a band of pipes and drums and "youths whose father and mother are still living" who carry banana plants. The boys are introduced to the banana plants. They are joined by their fathers, then by the mothers and elders. Sweets are distributed, signaling the beginning of prolonged dancing and singing. At three A.M., as the assemblage carries on its revelry, the male youths violently force their way into the house. There they engage in a mock battle with the father of the initiate. Some of these youths take a gourd and carry it some distance to a running stream or waterfall. One uses the gourd to scoop up living uncontaminated water that he must carry back to the ceremony, all the while being threatened by another youth with a spear. In another mock battle, they force their way back into the circumcision house where they fill the special gourd with the "powerful" water from the waterfall.

The circumcision takes place at dawn. The child's grandmother, to prepare for his entry into the house, dances a last dance. The path leading to the house is scattered with cattle dung, and a rice mortar is placed on the threshold, also covered with dung. (Cattle dung is a sign of wealth in Merina society.) As the moment for cutting approaches, the men in the house walk outside and form a semicircle in front of the entry. The women remain inside. The boy is handed to his grandfather, who sits in the dung-covered rice mortar. One of the elders then takes the special gourd and pours the powerful water over the child's penis, saying, as he does so, "May you be strong! May you be rich! May you have possessions! May you have cattle! May you have seven boys and seven girls!" Subsequently, the circumciser rubs the child's wound with a thick black paste to promote healing. Meanwhile, after the water has been poured on the child, one of the elders pitches the gourd some distance away. This sets off a melee, men and women scrambling and shoving, tearing at the gourd, trying to snatch a piece of it. These pieces are believed to convey fertility to their holders, and villagers place them under their beds. The boy, timorous and tearful, is picked up and passed to his mother through the window of the house. Tribal lore proscribes handing an uncircumcised boy through a window owing to the belief that, if this occurs, his penis will be unable to penetrate a woman's vagina and he will be unable to consummate his marriage. The mother is given a chicken to cook for the boy. After a few weeks some of the family may reconvene for a special meal to celebrate the healing of the wound.

When Bloch first observed this ceremony, one aspect caught him off guard. No sooner was the surgery finished than the circumciser handed the child's prepuce to an older male relative, who sandwiched it in a small piece of banana and ate it. Modern medicine's view has been that the foreskin is useless; after the operation it is discarded. Ritual circumcision, in contrast, in Madagascar and many other places, holds the foreskin in talismanic esteem. Its disposal is tied inextricably to its meaning. Many tribes bury it, sometimes simply in the dry earth, sometimes covered by soil bloodied during the operation, and sometimes in an anthill so that the earth's tiny scavengers may reclaim it and prevent it from being used for evil purposes. Some aboriginal tribes in Australia hide dried foreskins in secret spots invested with sacred energy: rocks, hollow trees, caves, and other totem places. In other tribes, the prepuce is presented to a sister of the initiate, who dries it, daubs it with red ochre and wears it on a string necklace. During the 1920s among the Ait Yusi in Morocco, one writer noted that at the end of the ritual, the foreskin was presented to the boy's mother, who attached it to a little stick taken from her spindle, placed this on her head and danced about with it. After the dance, she hung the prepuce over the top of her family's tent for a week before finally discarding it.[16]

Eighteenth-century French naturalist and historian Georges de Buffon reported that Persian women swallowed their sons' foreskins to ensure fertility. Several travelers commented on Australian tribes' habit of roasting the severed prepuce over a fire and presenting it to the boy's mother. The Hova were said either to give it to the circumcised boy's father or, failing that, to wrap it inside a banana leaf and feed it to a calf. In some areas of Mali, the Dogon grind severed foreskins with millet and mold the mixture into small cakes that are eaten by the circumcised themselves on the third day after the ritual. In other villages among the same tribe, the prepuces (and amputated clitorises from female circumcisions) are buried in rat holes, burned, or tossed into garbage piles.[17]

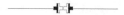

While early anthropologists labored to describe the tribal rites they encountered around the world, circumcision also attracted the notice of Sigmund Freud and his followers. They saw it as powerful, mystical, and hard to fit into any larger explanatory framework. Its importance was beyond question. For those peoples who practiced ritual cutting, from the Jews to Australian aborigines, the surgery was anchored in the deepest recesses of their mythologies. Circumcision thus presented a natural target for psychoanalytic interpretation because it concerned the phallus, which, as an object both alluring and taboo, had become a Freudian fixation.

Freud developed the core psychodynamic and developmental insights that would beget psychoanalysis during the final years of the nineteenth century. Thereafter, at different stages in his career, he applied his theories wholesale, moving from individual cases to broad social and cultural criticism. As a Jew, Freud himself had been circumcised as an infant, though he subsequently left religious faith far behind. What intrigued him were connections between cutting the penis (as an anatomist of some learning, he did not consider the foreskin a separate structure) and his burgeoning theory of sexuality, including the relationship between childhood trauma and later neurosis.[18]

An apt student of his own heritage, Freud knew of Maimonides' opinion (shared widely within the rabbinic tradition) that circumcision was meant to be traumatic because its practical purpose was to inhibit male sexuality. He agreed that circumcision did indeed accomplish this, but unlike Maimonides he did not celebrate the result. By the mid-1890s he had become an advocate of vigorous sexual expression, convinced that physical or emotional repression of sexual arousal and release could provoke anxiety neurosis. "It is positively a matter of public interest," he warned, "that *men should enter upon sexual relation with full potency.*"[19]

Freud described a pattern of development in which children around the age of four or five years entered a "phallic" stage, enthralled by their genitals, and also afraid that something might happen to harm this marvelous organ. At the same time, according to Freud, boys experienced a strong Oedipal conflict, characterized by erotic impulses toward the mother and rivalry, typified by conscious or unconscious death wishes, with the father. As the child becomes aware of the differences between the external genitalia of males and females, castration anxiety becomes more acute. Jews and non-Jews, he wrote, perceived circumcision not just as painful but as the most primal threat. "Circumcision is the symbolical substitute of castration," he declared, "a punishment which the primeval father dealt his sons long ago out of the fullness of his power; and whosoever accepted this symbol showed by doing so that he was ready to submit to the father's will, although it was at the cost of a painful sacrifice." This idea became part of Freud's personal mythology and his speculation about a prehistoric past. Lecturing in Europe and America, he claimed that "in the early days of the human family, castration was performed on the growing boy by the jealous and cruel father, and that circumcision, which is so frequently an element in puberty rites, is an easily recognizable trace of it."[20]

This extravagant fantasy—that circumcision is symbolic castration, reinforcing the incest taboo—encouraged dozens of Freudians (mainly in the United States) to search for a universal theory of circumcision. Psychologist Theodore Reik construed circumcision as a kind of prospective punishment in which older members of the family or community chastised young males for their secret sexual desires. The anthropologist John Wesley Mayhew Whiting, as part of a larger theory connecting initiation rituals with child-rearing practices, said the trauma of circumcision was meant to break the incestuous bond between mother and son, easing the son's transition into a male world without inciting parricidal revolt against the father. In the quest for a unifying theme, however, these interpretations largely ignored circumcision's social and ritual significance. It was as though all the ritual and symbolism were merely incidental to a deeper psychological truth.[21]

Not that psychologists agreed about what this truth might be. Some, like Henry Nunberg in his book *Problems of Bisexuality as Reflected in Circumcision*

(1949), continued down the trail Freud had blazed. Nunberg asserted that the "study of the puberty rites of primitives proved that circumcision represents symbolic castration, its underlying motive being prevention of incest."[22] Based on psychoanalyses of his own patients, Nunberg concluded that boys who had been circumcised in infancy blamed what they felt was a castrating procedure on their mothers and, in consequence, harbored lingering feelings of hostility and guilt. Nunberg also viewed circumcision as an expression of deep-seated anxiety about gender. Removing the foreskin stood for removing the penis, he wrote, and this shedding of the penis permitted the male to become fe- malelike in his genitalia. Others took exactly the opposite view. Far from sym- bolizing castration, one psychoanalyst insisted, Jewish circumcision stemmed from "the wish to create in males a permanent erection of the penis to ensure . . . fertile sexuality and thence the continuity of the group."[23]

If their arguments are improbable, Freud and later proponents of a psy- choanalytic approach to circumcision nonetheless inspired their successors to investigate the psychological impact of the operation.

To explore the effects of circumcision on children in the so-called phallic state of development, for example, researchers at a mental hospital in Turkey conducted a study on twelve boys. Their method was to question each child's mother about his environment, emotional, social, and intellectual develop- ment, then to administer the Goodenough draw-a-man test, Rorschach blots, and CT scans to the children before and after surgery. They found that chil- dren seemed to regress, drawing themselves as smaller and younger than im- ages drawn earlier. "The operation is experienced by the child as an aggressive attack, with deadening implications," the authors concluded. "The results ob- tained for the different psychological tests indicate that circumcision is per- ceived by the child as an aggressive attack on his body, which damaged, mutilated and in some cases totally destroyed him. The feeling of 'I am now castrated' seems to prevail in the psychic world of the child." In this instance, the researchers were convinced that their findings bore out Anna Freud's hy- pothesis about childhood circumcision. A founder of child psychoanalysis, she had maintained that because children perceived no distinction between cir- cumcision and castration, an operation in childhood would strongly confirm the circumcised child's anxieties. The helplessness, deficiency, and physical shrinking of self-image observed in Turkey seemed to prove her right.[24]

The most ambitious attempt to find a transcendent psychological basis for circumcision was a treatise written in the early 1950s by the distinguished, and later notorious, psychotherapist Bruno Bettelheim, a self-styled Freudian who would become world famous for his interpretations of fairy tales and myths. "Whatever the origin and meaning of circumcision may be, it must originate in deep human needs," he wrote, "since it seems to have sprung up independently among many peoples, although in different forms." Moreover, even in places where the practice appears to have spread by diffusion, he reasonably noted, people would not lightly take up such a radical and risky operation. It was "a strange mutilation," all the stranger for its being "found among the most primitive and the most highly civilized people." Thus, he concluded, circumcision "must reflect profound needs."[25]

Bettelheim dismissed Freud's fable of primal castration. As he interpreted the evidence, circumcision reflected a deep-seated ambivalence about being confined to a single sex. "The desire to possess also the characteristics of the other sex is a necessary consequence of the sex differences," he suggested. But the actual fulfillment of this desire would mean losing one's own genitals, "hence the inexorable nature of castration anxiety in both sexes." Against this fear, the purpose of circumcision and other rites of initiation was not to exacerbate sexual anxiety but to palliate it. Accordingly, he contended that at the most basic level circumcision was not about castration. It was about fertility. *Symbolic Wounds: Puberty Rites and the Envious Male* (1954) bore a dedication to Freud, "whose theories," Bettelheim wrote, "gave us a fuller understanding of the mind of preliterate man." Against Freudian doctrine, however, the book proclaimed that "circumcision developed as a result both of man's desire to participate in the female power of procreation, and of woman's desire, if not to rob the male of the penis, at least to make him bleed from his genital as women do."[26]

Bettelheim's insights came partly from reading turn-of-the century accounts of Australian aborigines, above all Spencer and Gillen, and partly from interviewing his own patients. The latter were an unlikely source: mentally or emotionally disturbed children at the Sonia Shankman Orthogenic School of the University of Chicago. Blood fascinated the children, Bettelheim noticed, and some of them invested menstrual blood with magic powers. Circumcision and the bleeding it produced appealed to the children's imaginations because it seemed to promise that boys could possess magical powers equal to those of girls. Of these powers, the capacity to bear children was for Bettelheim's boys a profound source of envy. In a flight of fancy, he likened their attitude to Australian aboriginal circumcision rituals, in which boys are taken from their mothers, placed in seclusion among older men, and finally, through the initiation ritual, reborn as men. What the aboriginal ritual signified, he wrote, was that circumcision, with all its blood and pain, conferred on men the generative power of women. While they lack the power to produce babies, men, through the transforming circumcision ritual, demonstrate the power to produce men.

If there is a certain logic in such reasoning, ultimately Bettelheim's theories collapse into a pile of conflicting conjectures. Indeed, at the end of his study, he confessed: "There is much evidence that it is imposed or desired by women; but there is also much reason to believe that it is desired by men because (1) it makes them more male by freeing the glans, (2) it provides them with a sign of sexual maturity and with potent blood from the genital, and (3) it adds to their power by giving them symbolically the capabilities of women."[27]

Anthropologists generally spurned Bettelheim's interpretations. For one thing, the notion that the fantasies of psychotic children could illuminate complicated religious practices struck them as naïve and patronizing. Moreover, critics asked, if circumcision did in fact originate in something as fundamental as male envy of childbearing, why wasn't it universal? And why did many of the same groups that circumcised males also cut female genitalia?

Bettelheim missed what scholars in the field had long realized: namely, that among certain African groups—the Dogon, Bambara, the Lobi of Mali—cutting of male and female genitalia reflects their belief in the fundamental duality of human beings. In some tribes, a newborn is said to possess twin souls of both sexes. In girls, the masculine soul inhabits her clitoris, which is removed to free her to adopt a purely feminine identity. In boys, the female soul resides in the foreskin, so the ritual of circumcision is essential to masculinity. "After circumcision it is the man's duty to go after his lost femininity and find it again in his wife," explained social psychologist Pierre Erny in his study of African children. "And the woman who was freed from her masculinity at the time of excision finds it again in the person of her husband." Ethnographer Dominique Zahan writes of certain northwest African tribes: "In the spiritual realm the function of circumcision is still more nuanced. By circumcising man the blacksmith (who customarily performs the operation) takes away the 'femininity' from his spirit, that is, the cloudiness in his understanding, the wanzo." In the mythology of the tribes Zahan studied, wanzo is the agent of ignorance and spiritual pollution. It acts as spiritual gauze, veiling the mind, preventing a man from knowing himself and from knowing god. Self-knowledge and religious understanding depend on shedding the wanzo as a snake sheds its skin. A woman would only choose to marry a man who was free of wanzo. Yet because wanzo contains a male's feminine element, losing it deprives him of an essential ingredient of human being. Marriage thus reunites man with what he has lost in circumcision. Union and completeness is possible only through union with a woman.[28]

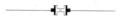

The appearance of circumcision in so many different cultures, ancient and modern, and infused with a bewildering variety of meanings has confounded attempts to construct a universal theory. No theory fits the myriad facts. No one has been able to identify a discrete biological or cultural predisposition for genital cutting. Perhaps, in this respect, the study of circumcision poses the same intellectual problem one sees more generally in ethnography. "Like poems and hypotheses," anthropologist Clifford Geertz observed, "ethnographies can only be judged *ex post*, after someone has brought them into being." And if ethnographic texts have any use at all, it is not to provide a single answer— not to isolate a universal element from the "trappings" of culture. Rather, it is, as Geertz suggests, to enable "conversations across societal lines—of ethnicity, religion, class, gender, language, race—that have grown progressively more nuanced, more immediate, and more irregular."[29] With a cultural practice as complicated as circumcision, as with Ibsen's onion in *Peer Gynt*, one can peel away layer after layer looking for the core without ever finding it. Indeed, to understand even one layer is difficult enough.

F O U R

From Ritual to Science

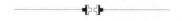

The operation of circumcision is one which may be performed for moral
reasons; one which is demanded for hygienic purposes; one which is frequently necessary for pathological conditions; and, finally, one which is of
unquestionably prophylactic importance.

—J. Henry C. Simes, "Circumcision" (1890)

ON THE RAINY MORNING OF FEBRUARY 9, 1870, A MANHATTAN DOCTOR NAMED
Lewis A. Sayre began his workday as usual, seated at his letter desk with a small
pot of tea. He was putting the finishing touches on a lecture about a new
treatment for lateral curvature of the spine. Absorbed in thought, the forty-
nine-year-old surgeon started when his servant bustled through the door and
handed him an envelope. He knew the handwriting at a glance. The message
came from an old friend, James Marion Sims, whose pioneering work in gynecology had earned him international fame. The previous afternoon, Sims
wrote, a wealthy couple from Milwaukee had shown up in his office begging
him to examine their young son. He obliged, but one look at the boy convinced him that he was seriously out of his depth. Could Sayre come at once?
Sims promised his colleague, "the little fellow has a pair of legs that you would
walk miles to see."[1]

Lewis Sayre was certainly the right person to call. In those days he was
America's leading orthopedic surgeon, a tall, solidly built man whose strong
nose, prominent brow, and square jaw framed by muttonchops projected com-
manding authority. Famously gifted with the scalpel, he was also a renowned
teacher and scholar, specializing in the anatomy of bones, joints, and muscles.

The discovery of a new musculoskeletal disease was as thrilling to him as the discovery of a new planet would be to an astronomer. So Sayre pushed his lecture aside, sent for his carriage and donned his overcoat.

On arriving at Dr. Sims's brownstone he was ushered immediately downstairs. There, in a small examination room, its walls scattered with medallions and ribbons that European royalty had bestowed on Sims, Sayre came face to face with "a most beautiful little boy of five years of age, but exceedingly white and delicate in his appearance." He was told that the child was "unable to walk without assistance or stand erect, his knees being flexed at about an angle of 45 degrees." Through the winter his condition had been worsening. Often the lad literally doubled up in pain. Finally, the parents, at their wits' end, had booked railroad passage to New York to seek the best treatment money could buy. Since the mother had once been Sims's patient and remained a lucrative source of referrals, he felt more than the usual obligation to do something for her son. Yet he could scarcely guess what was causing the boy's problem. Perhaps, he whispered to Sayre, in order to straighten the legs they should perform a tenotomy, the desperate remedy of cutting the child's hamstring tendons.[2]

After making his own physical examination, however, Sayre thought otherwise. "The deformity was due to *paralysis* and not *contraction*," he wrote, "and it was therefore *necessary to restore vitality to the partially paralyzed extensor muscles, rather than to cut the apparently contracted flexors*." In other words, the best solution lay in diagnosing the hidden source of paralysis and curing it. What made this case perplexing, however, was the absence of any visible injury to the legs or other symptoms of neurological disease.[3]

This was quite odd, but Sayre resolved to trace the malady to its source. With Sims's help, he proceeded to administer a battery of tests. One of these involved checking the boy's reflexes by applying electric current to his legs. While he was hooking up the wires, Sayre heard the child's nurse, who had been silently watching, exclaim, "Oh, doctor! Be very careful—don't touch his pee-pee—it's very sore." An examination of the genitals showed that the penis was normal, except that "the glans was very small and pointed, tightly imprisoned in the contracted foreskin, and in its efforts to escape, the meatus urinarius had become as puffed out and red as in a case of severe granular urethritis." Such inflammation was, the nurse said, a chronic condition. Often the pain kept the boy awake at night. Recently his penis had become so sensitive that even the slight friction of bedclothes caused painful erections.

Musing on the patient's history, Sayre had a flash of inspiration. Could the seemingly unrelated genital inflammation somehow be crippling the boy's legs? The more he thought about it, the more plausible the idea seemed. "As excessive venery is a fruitful source of physical prostration and nervous exhaustion, sometimes producing paralysis," he would later explain, "I was disposed to look upon this case in the same light, and recommended circumcision as a means of relieving the irritated and imprisoned penis."[4]

Here was a truly novel concept. So far as he knew, no one before had thought to use circumcision to cure paralysis. Nevertheless, with the mixture of instinct, confidence, and decisiveness that great surgeons must possess, Sayre grew so certain of his diagnosis that he had his coachman drive the boy directly to Bellevue Hospital, where he planned to demonstrate the operation to his medical students.

Early the next morning, the little patient chloroformed upon a marble table in the operating theater, Sayre drew the foreskin forward and cut it with scissors. To his surprise, "the mucous portion [remained] quite firmly adherent to the glans nearly to the orifice of the urethra." He had to improvise, finishing the procedure by "seizing the thickened mucous membrane with the thumbs and finger nails of each hand" and tearing it away from the glans. Whatever it lacked in elegance, this operation seemed to produce a wonderful result. Immediately after he awakened the child's health began to improve. Color returned to his cheeks. Soon he regained his appetite, slept soundly and, most remarkable of all, within a few weeks "was able to walk with his limbs quite straight." Astonishing as it seemed, Sayre proclaimed that circumcision, "simply quieting his nervous system by relieving his imprisoned glans penis," restored the patient to health.[5]

While the five-year-old was recuperating, the surgeon tried a similar experiment on the partially paralyzed son of a prominent New York attorney. This boy was older, in his teens, and barely able to walk. For more than a year Sayre had treated his paralysis with electric current, had "injected strychnia into the paralyzed muscles every tenth day," and had dosed him with iron and other tonics. Nothing had worked. Optimistic about his new hypothesis, Sayre recommended circumcision, maintaining that even if it didn't work, the procedure was unlikely to harm the lad. The worried father, who confided suspicion that his son "was guilty of masturbation," agreed without hesitation. Once again the outcome was miraculous. Shortly after the operation, Sayre reported, every symptom of paralysis vanished. Within a few weeks the lad recuperated so dramatically that "his most intimate friends scarcely recognize him."[6]

Medical breakthroughs often start with a single patient. Even though he had only a few cases to go on, Sayre convinced himself that genital irritation was the hidden culprit in many types of paralysis and hip-joint disease that stubbornly resisted standard treatments. Working in a busy New York City hospital, he had plenty of chances to test his theory. Several weeks later, in April 1870, he treated three young boys for crippling hip problems by detaching the foreskin from the glans penis. While it was not circumcision—the foreskin was left intact—"this slight operation," he wrote, "answered all the purposes of circumcision, and at once quieted their nervous irritability." These and other equally successful operations were enough to persuade him that he had unlocked the secret to a host of ills.

Sayre lost no time in publishing his findings in the *Transactions of the American Medical Association*. "Many of the cases of irritable children, with restless sleep, and bad digestion, which are often attributed to worms, is [*sic*] solely due to the irritation of the nervous system caused by an adherent or constricted prepuce," he asserted. "Hernia and inflammation of the bladder can also be produced by the severe straining to pass water in some of these cases of contracted prepuce." In times past, he told his fellow physicians, the medical literature had ignored the link between genital abnormalities, irritation, and disease. His duty was to make doctors aware of the facts; theirs in turn was to bring this new medical knowledge, and the best treatments, to their patients.[7]

A closer look suggests that Sayre's discovery was not quite as original as he claimed. Five years earlier, an English doctor named Nathaniel Heckford had published *Circumcision as a Remedial Measure in Certain Cases of Epilepsy, Chorea, etc.* (1865). This pamphlet derived from his work at the East London Hospital for Children (an institution he founded) where he had performed surgical experiments similar to Sayre's. Still, Heckford was a minor figure. His work attracted scant attention in England; his paper was never published in America.

Lewis Sayre, in contrast, sparked widespread interest on both sides of the Atlantic. This response was tribute not only to the surgeon's remarkable claims but also to his prominence and energy. The medical profession often presents its own history as a cavalcade of heroes. To his generation, as one medical historian put it, Sayre was a colossal figure, "philanthropist and missionary as well as surgeon."[8]

Proudly tracing his lineage to the *Mayflower*, Sayre had been a brilliant student, graduating in 1842 from New York's College of Physicians and Surgeons, then swiftly making a name for himself with a research paper on spinal irritation. While he liked research, he was practical to the fingertips. Early in his career, he would tell his son, "I made up my mind that if what I was taught agreed with my experience as to what I found, I would adopt it; otherwise not." Building a successful surgical practice among New York's affluent merchant class, Sayre at age thirty-three managed to get a surgical post at Bellevue Hospital. By 1859 his responsibilities had expanded to include the New York City Lunatic Hospital. When the Civil War broke out, the mayor named him resident physician for New York City. He used this position as a bully pulpit to campaign for sanitary reforms, including inspection of tenement housing, proper sewage disposal, and compulsory smallpox vaccination. In 1866 he sparked controversy by quarantining the steamer *Atlanta* in New York Harbor after hearing reports that cholera had broken out onboard. When the crisis passed, he was credited with saving the city from an outbreak of cholera like the awful epidemic of 1849. His professorship at Bellevue Medical College was the first chair in orthopedic surgery in the United States, and he used it as a platform for innovation. His *Lectures on Orthopedic Surgery and Disease of the Joints* (1876) went through a dozen editions and was the bible for a generation of surgeons. He was also an inventor, famous for designing a plaster-of-Paris body cast for straightening the spine. *Spinal Disease and Spinal Curvature* (1877), a book he produced to illustrate his various techniques and medical

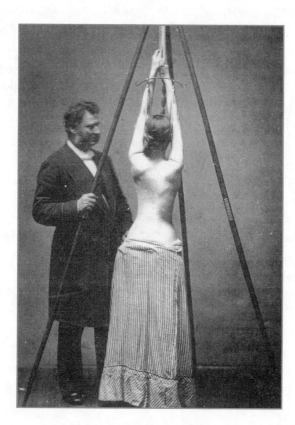

Lewis Sayre, shown here with a patient and a medical contraption he invented to treat curvature of the spine. From Lewis Sayre, *Spinal Disease and Spinal Curvature* (1877).

devices, became a classic, the first surgical monograph to feature mounted photographs of patients.[9]

Outside the operating room, he was a born organizer: the prime mover in the New York Pathological Society; an officer of the New York Academy of Medicine; and in 1866 vice president of the fledgling American Medical Association (AMA). In honor of his tireless striving on behalf of their profession, in 1880 the medical elite elected Lewis Sayre president of the AMA. One of Sayre's legacies was his campaign to upgrade the organization's published transactions, which he chose to rename *Journal of the American Medical Association*.

Lewis Sayre's great authority within his profession throws interesting light on why circumcision became widely accepted in American medicine. Medicine in mid-nineteenth-century America was, by all accounts, a mediocre profession. And doctors, in part because they were helpless against most serious diseases, were not highly respected. During the era of Reconstruction, however, the medical profession organized itself, with doctors becoming better educated, better organized and, in consequence, more hierarchical than they had been previously. A talented and charismatic man respected on both sides of the Atlantic, Sayre exemplified the rising professional order. "He has moved a great mass of painful, tedious and almost incurable complaints into the region of curable and easily managed affections," noted the *British Medical Journal*.[10] So when he insisted that serious orthopedic diseases could be cured by a fairly simple operation on the penis, the medical rank and file were prepared to take him seriously.

He championed his message with passion and persistence. For three decades, until his death in 1900, Sayre promoted circumcision in hundreds of speeches and papers, touting a wider and wider array of benefits. He used the operation to treat epilepsy, hernia, and a variety of mental disorders. In 1875 he published and distributed thousands of copies of a pamphlet, *Spinal Anemia with Partial Paralysis and Want of Co-operation from Irritation of the Genital Organs*, in which he argued that "peripheral irritation" from the foreskin sometimes caused "an insanity of the muscles," in which a victim's muscles acted "on their own account, involuntarily . . . without the controlling power of the person's brain."[11]

To illustrate his point, Sayre recounted the case of an eighteen-month-old boy he had recently treated. At first the baby raged out of control, "like a lunatic, an insane child," crying constantly, sleeping only when drugged with laudanum or morphine. Circumcision, boasted Sayre, produced "almost a miracle; it is beyond the power of man to comprehend it unless you see these cases from the start." Outcomes like this convinced him to try circumcision for chronic mental disorders, the most elusive of illnesses and hardest to treat.

Accompanied by two surgical assistants, Sayre and his scalpel made several excursions to nearby Manhattan State Hospital's Idiot Asylum on Randall's Island. There he examined the genitals of sixty-seven boys, attempting to establish a connection between genital irritation and imbecility. He operated on dozens of them. (Modern concepts of patients' rights and "informed consent" lay far in the future; Sayre saw no ethical problems in conducting his experiments.) Evaluating the research, he believed that some boys benefited. In the end, however, his research on lunacy and dementia ended in bitter disappointment. Despite the surgeries, no boy improved enough to be discharged from the asylum.[12]

Occasional setbacks failed to dampen Sayre's enthusiasm. Circumcision remained in his view a powerful and underused operation. He seldom missed a chance to promote it to his colleagues. Reprints of his articles and pamphlets were circulated at state and county medical society meetings all around the country. Owing to his illustrious orthopedic work, doctors flocked to his lectures. When he attended the great 1876 International Medical Congress in Philadelphia as an AMA delegate and gave a brilliant demonstration of hip-joint excision (of which Joseph Lister exclaimed, "This demonstration would of itself have been a sufficient reward for my voyage across the Atlantic"), Sayre took advantage of his platform to deliver a treatise titled *On the Deleterious Results of a Narrow Prepuce and Preputial Adhesion.*[13]

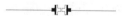

That various diseases were caused by abnormalities in the foreskin and thus could be treated by its removal was an idea that fit the times. Surgeons in the 1870s aggressively operated on the genitalia of both sexes for all kinds of complaints. How the sexual organs influenced physical and mental health was an ancient question, predating Hippocrates by centuries. Yet in the Victorian era, the mystery seemed solvable based on a theory known as *reflex neurosis.*

Every age has its own metaphors for the body. During the last decades of the nineteenth century, most educated doctors pictured the human body as an intricate web of nervous affinity radiating through the spine into each organ. The heart, the liver, the kidneys, the sexual organs—each was thought to possess its own spheres of neural influence, governing different aspects of body and mind. And each was wired, however indirectly, to every other. In some ways reflex neurosis resembles the theory behind acupuncture: a whole human being interconnected by a complex system of channels, so that a minor agitation or blockage in one part of the body might crop up in a seemingly unrelated area.

Reflex neurosis theory attributed many diseases to "irritation." Biologists supposed that the nervous system, organs, tissues, and later, even cells could be disturbed by friction so slight as to be undetectable. The idea of irritation was taken to its extreme when the pioneering cell biologist Rudolf Virchow speculated that irritation was the root cause of malignant tumor growth. Cancers, which seemed to come from nowhere, in Virchow's opinion resulted from infinitesimal cellular friction. To him, along with many others, the basic appeal of irritation and reflex neurosis theories was that cryptic disorders such as depression and neurasthenia, as well as cancer, had a discrete somatic basis. If a specific irritation could be traced back to its source, presumably it could also be eradicated and the patient cured.[14]

This was an exciting prospect—and it greatly encouraged the use of exploratory surgery. Based on reflex neurosis theory, for example, American gynecologists, led by Sayre's friend James Marion Sims, devised scores of experimental genital surgeries to alleviate psychological abnormalities in women.

Cutting the body to heal the mind could produce appalling results. One young Georgia surgeon, Robert Battey, gained notoriety for inventing the so-called normal ovariotomy. Convinced that once a woman had borne children her sexual organs were superfluous and a potential source of disease, he removed women's healthy ovaries to alleviate symptoms ranging from hysteria and neurasthenia to backache. Battey's operation, accepted on both sides of the Atlantic, was especially popular in America where, according to one historian, it "was not a marginal procedure conducted by a handful of crackpots, but central in the arsenal of late-nineteenth-century gynecology."[15]

Many other doctors (including Sayre) were sure that the best cure for female "nervousness"—a catchall diagnosis for anything from insomnia to depression—was clitoridectomy. Obviously the clitoris was extremely sensitive; in some women it seemed to become hypersensitive, triggering a host of ailments. It became a prime suspect in cases involving nonspecific symptoms and so was subjected to numerous surgeries, manipulations, and chemical concoctions.[16]

In theory, reflex neurosis applied equally to males and females. Both sexes appeared to have similar nervous systems and to be subject to similar organic disturbances, including pelvic or genital irritations, that might provoke physical or mental disease. Equally important, men and women both were subject to the peculiar stresses of the American environment. "Persons who are very sensitive nervously, and especially Americans, living in our American climate, are liable to develop all or many of the symptoms of sexual neurasthenia," wrote George Beard, a New York authority on nervous disorders. Like many of his colleagues, Beard thought that American men were especially prone to nervous breakdown, and that genital irritation was a major factor.[17]

In men who exhibited "a temperament previously made sensitive by exhausting climate, work, worry, tobacco, alcohol" and other excesses, genital irritation could incite a dangerous downward spiral. Circumcision was only one of a dozen treatments Beard used to break the grip of disease. Usually he preferred to begin with electricity.

> Electricity may be applied to the male genital organs in various ways, and by both currents—galvanic and faradic.
>
> *First.*—One electrode in the rectum and the other in the urethra, both insulated nearly to their tips. In this method *very mild* currents must be used . . .
>
> *Second.*—One insulated electrode in the rectum and the other . . . between the penis and the scrotum, or over the pubis, and on the inner side of thighs. In this method very strong currents can be used.
>
> *Third.*—One pole connected with an uninsulated sound in the urethra, and the other on the thighs or on the spine. Strong currents can be borne in this method also. In this method the mechanical effect of the sound is combined with the special effect of the electricity. I have devised a special clamp for connecting the electricity with the sounds.
>
> *Fourth.*—Purely external applications, one electrode pressed firmly on the scrotum, the other on the spine or the back of the neck, or on the inner sides of the thighs, the nerves of which affect reflexively to the general apparatus in a powerful way. . . .
>
> *Sixth.*—Drawing off sparks on the spine and the genital region by statical electricity (franklinization).

Ghastly as Beard's regimen sounds, electric current was the technology of choice for sexual dysfunction in men or nervous disorders suspected of originating in genital irritation.

Apart from traditional urology—relieving obstructions, removing diseased tissue, and so forth—sexual surgery on men was comparatively rare. While it seemed permissible for male surgeons to use the scalpel heroically on women's pelvic organs, undeterred by the prospect of "unsexing" their patients, they applied different standards on male patients. Few surgeons wanted to risk impotence unless they clearly confirmed life-threatening symptoms. Moreover, even if they had tried to expand sexual surgery on men, it is unlikely that surgeons would have overridden patients' objections. In a culture that discounted female sexuality, doctors found women more submissive than men to the dictates of medical authority.

Yet while clitoredectomy and Battey's operation fell out of favor, circumcision became standard practice. Even in the days of their greatest acceptance, sexual surgeries were performed on only a small minority of women. In contrast, circumcision was quietly democratized, and ultimately extended to most of America's male population.

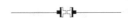

The procedure's first medical advocates were physicians who followed the lead of Lewis Sayre. They circumcised to cure disease. Before long, though, these men were joined by other doctors who insisted that circumcision would benefit any male, whether or not he presented symptoms or abnormalities. Arguing that an ounce of prevention was worth a pound of cure, they constructed a rationale for prophylactic surgery.

Cutting a normal, healthy patient to prevent disease in the future was unprecedented. It was obvious to surgeons that the scalpel presented a grave insult to the body. Operations were seen as an evil justified only if they averted a greater evil. Hence, Hippocrates' famous dictum *primum non nocere* (first, do no harm) advised physicians to avoid any treatment likely to leave the patient worse off.

Generally, practitioners relied on the principle of medical necessity in deciding whether or not to operate. In the case of circumcision, the time-honored medical indications were cancerous lesions and phimosis, a painful constriction of the foreskin that interfered with normal function. In cases like these, cutting was plainly justified. But such cases were uncommon. Phimosis severe enough to warrant surgery was so unusual that doctors considered it a rare disease. Penile cancer was rarer still; few doctors ever saw a case. Medical textbooks and professional journals, when they mentioned disorders of the penis at all, passed over them cursorily.

Perceptions began to change, though, when Lewis Sayre, based on the concept of reflex neurosis, alerted physicians to suspect genital irritation or phimosis when they were confronted by confusing, seemingly unrelated symptoms. Before the distinguished surgeon sounded the alarm, wrote a leading Georgia doctor, "*congenital phimosis* and *adherent prepuce*, as a cause of paralysis, reflex muscular contraction, curvature of the spine and acquired deformity, escaped the notice of the profession." Whereas doctors had always considered phimosis a *local* ailment, Sayre characterized it as *systemic*: a perpetual state of excitement, erection, and nervous irritation radiating dangerously throughout the body. As the first doctor to formulate this theory, according to his peers, he deserved "the credit of waking the profession up upon this condition of the genital apparatus." Once he had established "the reflex nervous consequences of genital irritation," noted an admiring editorial in the *Louisville Medical News*, physicians around the country began to confirm his observations with accounts of their own cases.[18]

Hence one Louisville doctor, unable to relieve an infant's spasms and high fever, tried circumcising him. Two days later the baby recovered. In Philadelphia, E. P. Hurd reported examining a five-month-old who suffered from whooping cough, chronic crying, and unexplained weight loss. Upon finding that "our infantile sufferer revealed a sadly neglected phimosis," Hurd cut away his foreskin, a procedure whose delicacy he likened to resecting "the femur of a grasshopper." Before the operation, urine specimens had contained "a copious sediment of uric acid [and] crystalline structures." Shortly afterward this "lithuria" disappeared, leading Hurd to conclude that irritation from the foreskin must somehow have been impairing the baby's kidney function. Since theory held that phimosis could short-circuit the nervous system, it occurred to J. A. Hofheimer to operate on a youth of eighteen who had been epileptic since birth. For years he had averaged one to three seizures a week. Circumcision immediately reduced the frequency of the attacks to "sometimes only one in two or three months," the doctor wrote. "Four years have elapsed since the operation and his condition continues to improve."[19]

Before the development of controlled clinical studies, no one thought to ask whether the case histories that proliferated in medical journals were biased toward success, reflecting only good results. Yet it is plain that writers had little incentive to broadcast their failures. Organized medicine is far more interested in discovering what works than ferreting out what doesn't. The annals of failed experiments remain unpublished. The result of the professional preference for good news was to make it seem to readers of medical journals that circumcision was remarkably effective for a long list of complaints.

And the list kept growing. Every month, it seemed, writers found new ailments associated with phimosis and "adherent prepuce," a label they used to describe virtually any problem with the foreskin. In modern terms, doctors were learning to associate the foreskin with certain risk factors for disease. But how were they to apply these new ideas in the clinic? For a start, except at the extremes they lacked clear guidelines for distinguishing what was healthy from what was abnormal and potentially harmful. What was the expected range of normal human variation? And if the organ did present some abnormality, how should one decide whether to treat it or leave it alone? In most parts of the country, medical education was notoriously haphazard. When it came to sex, few physicians knew in accurate detail how the male organ ordinarily developed from infancy to maturity. Even among experts—urology specialists and medical school professors—the complex anatomy of the penis was poorly understood.

Though often unsure exactly what they should be looking for, physicians began routinely to examine baby boys' genitals. The closer they looked, the more worried they became. Few babies appeared perfectly sound. Almost all boys younger than three or four years exhibited some degree of adherent prepuce. (Ordinarily, the foreskin does not separate from the penis and become fully retractable until around the age of ten.) If adherent prepuce endangered a baby's health, most boys seemed to be at risk.

As doctors checked more carefully for abnormalities, the perceived incidence of phimosis grew apace. In a typical medical paper, Norman H. Chapman, a disciple of Sayre's who served as professor of nervous and mental disease at the University of Kansas City, declared that while no one could tabulate the rate of congenital phimosis, it was undoubtedly much greater than people suspected. Even when there was no phimosis, he advised, since a long and contracted foreskin was so often a source of "secondary complications . . . it is always good surgery to correct this deformity . . . as a precautionary measure, even though no symptoms have as yet presented themselves." In this regard, he felt that Christians stood to learn something from Jews. "Moses was a good sanitarian," Chapman reasoned, "and if circumcision was more generally practised at the present day, I believe that we would hear far less of the pollutions and indiscretions of youth; and that our daily papers would not be so profusely flooded with all kinds of sure cures for loss of manhood."[20]

Chapman wrote these words in 1882, and his language illustrates an inflection point in medical opinion. Here was a distinguished physician advocating circumcision not primarily to eliminate reflex irritation, but more broadly as a preventive, hygienic measure that would contribute to public health.

New reasons for the procedure were certainly important if it were to gain wider acceptance because reflex neurosis theory, long questioned in some circles, was coming under increasing assault. That Sayre performed his operations and some patients got better hardly proved the theory. What about the boys who didn't recover? As early as 1881, in a direct attack on Sayre, a Brooklyn doctor named Langdon C. Gray flatly told the New York Neurological Society that "in not one of the cases of reflex paralysis supposed to be dependent upon genital irritation, which have thus far been published, is there conclusive proof of this relation of cause and effect." Implicitly, however, even a physician who had misgivings about reflex neurosis theory and might never have considered using circumcision to treat paralysis could endorse circumcision as a sanitary reform.[21]

This was precisely the reasoning of doctors such as J. M. McGee. Enthusiastic after reading Sayre's first papers, he had tried to produce similar miracles with paralyzed children in his own practice. But to his "sad disappointment" his first efforts at cutting the prepuce effected no cures. Still he persisted, and in further trials was elated to find that circumcision could have unanticipated effects. A boy with a bad case "of tubercular meningitis was temporarily rendered less irritable, slept better, etc. One of myetitis . . . showed 'marked improvement.' One of *brass poisoning* completely cured!" No scientific theory explained these remarkable outcomes. Indeed, McGee frankly confessed his bewilderment. Still, a doctor's first obligation was to his patient, he decided, and he felt duty-bound to promote anything that worked, whether or not he understood why.

Whether it be curative or not it is conservative, and removes one source of irritation from an exquisitely sensitive organ. I would favor circumcision, however, independent of existing disease, as a sanitary precaution. . . . (1.) The exposure of the glans to friction, etc., hardens it, and renders it less liable to abrasion in sexual intercourse, and consequently venereal ulcer. (2.) It is acknowledged to be useful as a preventive of masturbation. (3.) It certainly renders the accident of phymosis and paraphymosis impossible. (4.) It prevents the retention of sebaceous secretion and consequent balanitis. (5.) It probably promotes continence by diminishing the pruriency of the sexual appetite. And its performance surely settles forever the question of reflex trouble as to that particular cause.[22]

Circumcision, in a word, made the patient cleaner.

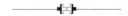

Yet "sanitary precaution," as McGee called it, is more complicated than it may appear. In every age, in every culture, conceptions of clean and dirty are heavily loaded with moral, social, and cultural meanings. A classic approach to unriddling these connotations has been suggested by the historical study of manners, habits, and personal comportment. Inspired by Norbert Elias's groundbreaking book *Ueber den Prozess der Zivilisation* (1939; translated into English as *The Civilizing Process* in 1978), scholars such as Lawrence Wright and Richard L. Bushman have delved into behaviors so commonplace—spitting, farting, bathing, and so forth—that they scarcely seemed historically significant.[23]

The "civilizing process" originated in European courts during the sixteenth century as sets of increasingly elaborate rules or "manners" by which people learned to check their natural bodily impulses. Little by little, in France and elsewhere, people admitted into the presence of royalty were expected to show respect through conspicuous restraint. Over the centuries, more and more behaviors became subject to the discipline of manners, first for members of the court, then gradually for the upper and middle classes who sought to emulate courtly demeanor. To Elias's Freudian way of thinking, this apparent march of progress also had its dark side. The body was reined in at the price of freedom and spontaneity. Too much control, too many rules, repressed natural urges. The result was neurosis, the discontent of the civilized. The ultimate tragedy of modernity was that, in the process of observing proper decorum, people became alienated from their own bodies.

There is a modern assumption that, beyond any other cultural or religious significance it may have had, since the time of the ancient Egyptians circumcision must always have served an essentially hygienic purpose. But this assumption was not part of American or European thinking until the 1880s, when a generation of doctors decided that the circumcised penis was more sanitary than uncircumcised. They arrived at this view at a time when Americans were making major efforts to clean up the urban environment and, not incidentally, were also developing new standards of personal cleanliness. In early nineteenth-century America, people seldom bathed. This changed in the decades after the Civil War, when scrubbing with soap became a routine for millions of citizens who considered personal hygiene evidence of social and cultural refinement. Among Americans, changes in bathing habits were part of a cultural transformation rooted in a deep-seated yearning for superior cultivation and gentility. Cleansing with soap, brushing one's hair, clipping one's nails, and other acts of personal grooming literally separated the washed from the unwashed.[24]

Americans gave a new twist to John Wesley's saying that cleanliness is next to godliness. They identified being clean with good morals, sound health, and upright character. Countless pamphlets and dime novels placed a bathtub at the beginning of the path that led a boy from rags to riches. Unsanitary meant corrupt, Victorian moralist William A. Alcott reminded his readers, adding that "he who neglects his person and dress will be found lower in the scale of morals, other things being equal, than he who pays a due regard to cleanliness."[25]

Alcott and his contemporaries did not hesitate to apply this logic expansively. During the Gilded Age, an era obsessed with racial and social hierarchies, writers commonly ranked entire civilizations, peoples, and social groups from clean to dirty. In the eyes of the growing middle class, according to one historian, "cleanliness indicated control, spiritual refinement, breeding; the unclean were vulgar, coarse, animalistic." To be sufficiently clean, in other words, became a basic standard of social virtue. Dirt was a moral and thus a social hazard whose stigma people would strive painstakingly to avoid.[26]

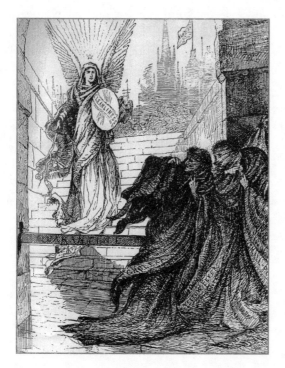

The angel of cleanliness, armed with sword and shield, stands at the gate of New York. The contagious diseases huddled below are drawn to suggest immigrants. *Harper's Weekly* (1885).

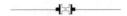

Although the new-fashioned cultural significance of cleanliness helps explain the popular acceptance of genital hygiene, it doesn't explain why, for instance, surgery should have replaced soap and water. After all, other industrial nations at different times adopted higher standards of personal cleanliness without taking up circumcision. Outside Anglo-American medicine, improved hygiene meant washing more thoroughly and more often. (How thoroughly and how often was, and remains to this day, a matter of considerable national variation.) The extraordinary medical transformation of circumcision in America—and to a lesser extent in England, where Lewis Sayre also lectured, published, and was in 1877 decorated by the British Medical Association—was inspired by a peculiar new vision of what was clean and what was dirty.

At the heart of this new vision was the greatest intellectual breakthrough in nineteenth-century medicine: the germ theory of disease.

In Wollstein, Germany, an intrepid surgeon and medical researcher named Robert Koch electrified the medical community by identifying microscopic bacteria that caused a number of terrible infectious diseases: anthrax (1876), tuberculosis (1882), conjunctivitis, and cholera (1883). Appointed to direct the hygienic institute at Berlin, Koch continued for the rest of his long life to hunt down microbes for dread diseases such as malaria and bubonic plague. Meanwhile, even better known in the United States, the celebrated French chemist Louis Pasteur crusaded for a series of public health measures based on the theory that bacilli, invisible to the naked eye, brought about most virulent and contagious infections.

The majestic discoveries of Koch and Pasteur and the new science of bacteriology they championed were trumpeted in the popular and professional press. Inevitably, the way in which doctors and the public pictured contagion changed. People readily understood the image of microbes as tiny living agents of contagion that could be transmitted from person to person. Still, practical applications were limited; the notion that invisible bacteria spawned diseases like tuberculosis was hard to translate into new ways of treating patients. It is one thing to identify an infectious microbe, and quite another to invent a vaccine or drug to vanquish it. Consequently, germ theory, at least as far as clinical practice was concerned, created bafflement within the medical community. Before the invention of sulfa compounds and antibiotic drugs such as penicillin in the 1930s and 1940s, the most effective and popular uses of germ theory were in preventive medicine.[27]

Few doctors had enough training in basic science to understand new biological research. Fewer still had any idea how it might apply to individual patients or to public health. More than a generation after the discovery of germ theory, when a violent epidemic of polio swept America on the eve of World War I, doctors were bewildered and almost completely powerless to deal with the crisis. Viruses, in contrast to bacteria, had not yet been characterized. Yet even though the mechanism behind polio and its means of transmission was not understood, public health officials resolved to act forcefully. They cobbled together policies based on sanitation, personal hygiene, and quarantine of infected patients. Their efforts had little effect, and the epidemic ran its course. Stymied by an enigmatic disease, doctors relied on whatever tools were at hand, not pausing to verify whether or not their methods actually worked.[28]

Lacking effective treatments or a real understanding of how microbes were transmitted, many physicians considered surgery a potent weapon against infection. With characteristic zeal, a Rhode Island health official named Charles V. Chapin reminded his peers of the potential epidemiological benefits of the operations they performed. If they really wanted to halt the spread of childhood diseases, he announced, it was "more important to remove adenoids from the child than it is to remove ashes from the back yard." Acting in the spirit of Chapin's suggestion, public health physicians in New York briefly tried removing the gall bladders of carriers of typhoid fever because they were thought to carry infectious bacteria.[29]

Germ theory ignited germ phobia. The press popularized an image of the human body as a conveyance for all sorts of hazardous microbial agents. Newspapers and magazines in the Gilded Age displayed a prurient fixation on the dirt associated with bodily functions: excrement, urine, blood, pus, and other secretions. Being closely identified with "dirty" waste products of the body, the genitals were often found filthy by association. Obviously they produced unpleasant substances. Worse, they were channels for sexually transmitted diseases.

With such thoughts in mind, around 1890 medical writers drifted into the habit of portraying the penis itself as a source of contamination. Using a term formerly reserved for contagious diseases, for instance, a St. Louis physician named Jonathan Young Brown went so far as to label smegma—thick sebaceous secretions that collect beneath the foreskin—"infectious material."[30] (Ironically, Brown appears not to have realized that the word *smegma* derived from Greek and Latin words for cleansing and soap.) If the foreskin harbored this bacteria-laden substance, it followed that circumcision, by eliminating it, could be considered preventive medicine, a safeguard against infection. Logic seemed to dictate removing the prepuce routinely—cleaning up the penis—as a prudent matter of public health.

This principle found its champion in Peter Charles Remondino, a physician and public health official practicing on the West Coast. Like Lewis Sayre, Remondino was hyperactive within his profession—vice president of the California Medical Society, an official of the Southern California chapter of American Public Health Association, and a prolific writer of letters and papers.

In the early 1880s he stumbled across Sayre's work and was deeply impressed by its sound reasoning and amazing results. The distinguished surgeon, he wrote, was "the Columbus of the prepuce," the scientific explorer who charted "this territory [that] Hippocrates and Galen overlooked." Fascinated by an operation so simple yet seemingly so rich in benefit, and eager to broadcast the good news to a wider audience, Remondino spent several years scouring libraries to research his magnum opus, *History of Circumcision* (1891). Despite its title, the book is less history than polemic. The author knew that while patients could be talked into surgery when they suffered injury or distress, "such a thing as surgery to remedy a seemingly medical disease, or what might be called the preventive practice of surgery, is something they cannot understand." He wrote to change their minds. For more than three hundred closely printed pages, he ransacked world history, piling up a mountain of evidence "to furnish my professional brothers with some embodied facts that they may use in convincing the laity . . . that circumcision is absolutely necessary."[31]

To a modern reader, Remondino's so-called facts are a rambling, slapdash collection of folklore, conjecture, and pseudo-science. No more a scientist than he was a historian, he had absorbed just enough of Darwin to surmise that the foreskin was a vestige of man's evolutionary past. Naked savages might have needed foreskins for protection as they scampered through the brambles. "With improvement in man's condition and his gradual evolution into a higher sphere," Remondino confidently insisted, "the prepuce became a superfluity." And a treacherous one at that.

> The prepuce seems to exercise a malign influence in the most distant and apparently unconnected manner; where, like some of the evil genii or sprites in the Arabian tales, it can reach from afar the object of its malignity, striking him down unawares in the most unaccountable manner; making him a victim to all manner of ills, sufferings, and tribulations; unfitting him for marriage or the

cares of business; making him miserable and an object of continual scolding and punishment in childhood, through its worriments and nocturnal enuresis; later on, beginning to affect him with all kinds of physical distortions and ailments, nocturnal pollutions, and other conditions calculated to weaken him physically, mentally, and morally; to land him, perchance, in jail or even in a lunatic asylum. Man's whole life is subject to the capricious dispensations and whims of this Job's-comforts-dispensing enemy of man.

Born with "this unyielding tube," 95 percent of uncircumcised men, he guessed, suffered from some degree of phimosis. While Remondino accepted Sayre's hypothesis about reflex irritation at face value, he was prepared to go much further, arguing that the most common diseases associated with the foreskin were not matters of reflex neurosis at all. These included rheumatic complaints, asthma, Bright's disease and other renal disorders, and more ominously, impotence, penile cancer, and syphilis. Considering the magnitude of its dangers, he proclaimed, "life-insurance companies should class the wearer of the prepuce under the head of hazardous risks."[32]

Few of Remondino's findings were original. The connection between cancer and the foreskin, for example, for years had been a matter of concern. In 1878, in his standard treatise on surgery, John Ashurst, Professor of Clinical Surgery at the University of Pennsylvania, said that phimosis made men more susceptible to venereal infections and predisposed them "to the development of malignant disease." Among regular doctors in the 1880s and 1890s, the most popular explanations for cancer held (following Virchow's theory) that it was "excited," as Sir Herbert Snow claimed, by "some continued mechanical irritant." Different organs of the body responded to particular irritants. Common sense suggested that venereal lesions like chancre were prime sites for cancerous irritation. There was no doubt that the foreskin itself was occasionally a target of infection and that circumcised men rarely if ever suffered from penile cancer. Indeed, this disorder was virtually unknown among Jews. Although its incidence among Gentiles was exceedingly low, its effects were hideous. Any physician who saw a case remembered it vividly. By the end of the century, although no scientist had been able to figure out the precise etiology of the disease, surgeons took it for granted that irritation from the foreskin, even in the absence of any infection, was "a predisposing cause to epithelioma of the penis."[33]

Circumcision as a precaution against malignancy was appealing, for Victorians, like their descendants a century later, lived in dread of cancer. The awful public ordeal of President Ulysses S. Grant, who died an agonizing death from what his doctors diagnosed as "an epithelioma" of the soft palate, transfixed the public and the medical community alike. Autopsy findings convinced Grant's physicians that his disease had been caused by irritation, specifically irritation in the mouth and throat from years of puffing cigars. Epithelioma, one of Grant's doctors explained, "as a rule starts from local irritation, and unlike other forms of cancer, is not dependent upon hereditary disposition to the disease." Penile cancers were believed to grow along similar lines. In fact, the mucosal tissue lining the inside of the prepuce bore a close resemblance to the tissue inside the mouth. In a world with no effective weapon against malignancies, the view that "the prepuce is the inciting cause as well as the initial point of attack" became an accepted reason to operate before cancer struck.[34]

Venereal infections, owing to their contagiousness and social stigma, were feared as much as cancer. Syphilis in particular raged out of control, approaching epidemic proportions in America's urban centers. During the 1880s and 1890s, medical researchers, taking their lead from Koch and Pasteur, made great strides in understanding the pathology of syphilis and gonorrhea. Therapeutics, however, lagged dismayingly behind. Laboratories produced no magic bullet. The virtues of chastity, widely celebrated in rhetoric, were unpopular in practice. Well into the twentieth century physicians continued to dose patients with mercury and experiment with compounds more likely to poison them than palliate their disease.[35]

Given their lack of effective resources to treat sexually transmitted diseases, physicians' belief that circumcision provided prophylaxis is perhaps understandable. In his treatise on surgery, John Ashurst told medical students that the prepuce makes men "more liable to various forms of venereal infection, and becomes a serious complication when venereal diseases are acquired." A Chicago surgeon, A. C. Williams, reported that of the more than 400 circumcisions he had performed, at least half had been done to cure genital herpes. "Many men who have herpes," he wrote, "imagine they have syphilis, and with or without the advice of a physician take constitutional treatment" like toxic mercury compounds. "I would follow in the footsteps of Moses and circumcise all male children." J. Henry C. Simes, Professor of Genito-Urinary and Venereal Disease in the Philadelphia Polyclinic, noting that venereal diseases were markedly less prevalent in Jews than Gentiles, agreed. Circumcision, he reasoned, "causes the epithelial covering to become more of the nature of the skin rather than that of the mucous membrane," and therefore repellent to venereal microorganisms.[36]

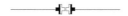

If circumcision reduced men's risk of infection, it stood to reason that Jews should be healthier than Gentiles. Strong evidence for such a view emerged in the form of an epidemiological study on the health of American Jews published in 1890 and summarized the following year in the distinguished *North American Review.* "On the Vital Statistics of the Jews," written by the eminent physician John S. Billings, drew on data from the 1880 Census to sketch an unexpected portrait. "Death-rates of this race are lower," Billings observed; "they have fewer still-born children, greater average longevity, and [are] less liable to certain forms of disease than other races." He reported, for example, that the incidence of cancer among Jews was low: 6.48 per 1,000, compared to 10.01 per 1,000 for the general population. Also, the much-maligned defective classes—insane, idiots, epileptics—were far less prevalent among Jews than among the Gentile majority. At a time when public health officials were desperate to slow the spread of disease among newly arrived immigrants, Billings's work inspired scores of studies focused on learning why Jews, even in the poorest ghettos, enjoyed favorable rates of morbidity and mortality.[37]

To many leading physicians, the possibility that circumcision protected Jews from certain diseases quickly became certitude, especially when new research confirmed that the incidence of penile epithelioma and syphilis among Jews was strikingly lower than among Gentiles.[38] Jewish physicians, whose attitudes toward circumcision were shaped by their own culture and experience, found this evidence especially compelling. "Judaism has made religion the handmaid of science," wrote a leading Jewish doctor and public health researcher. "It has utilized piety for the preservation of health." Carrying this thought to a bizarre extreme, Peter Remondino asserted that circumcision itself "is the real cause of the differences in longevity and faculty for enjoyment of life that the Hebrew enjoys in contrast to his Christian brother."[39]

Had they looked beyond physiology to Jewish culture and social organization, turn-of-the-century researchers would have found more plausible clues to the population's good health. The incidence of syphilis, for instance, surely had less to do with either heredity or circumcision than with how Jewish patterns of sexual activity differed from those of other ethnic groups.

Emulating an ancient ritual that involved cutting the penis might have seemed a strange innovation for a country devoted to its identity as a Christian nation. Yet there is abundant evidence that American Christians were usually quite tolerant of Judaism and its rituals. In 1867, for example, when a San

Francisco pawnbroker named Henry Danziger announced that he was the father of three newborn boys—the first triplets born in the West—their circumcision ceremony turned into the social event of the season. The boys' bris
attracted a well-heeled crowd of Jews and Gentiles, the latter, according to the
Hebrew Observer, seeming "to take a lively interest in this . . . altogether novel
ceremony." If the *Observer* found any reason for complaint, it was that the
ladies who packed the balcony of the synagogue took *too* lively an interest in
the procedure.

> We are decidedly opposed to such a gathering of females, both old and young,
> on similar demonstrations [and] it strikes us as altogether out of taste for ladies
> to bend over the galleries to witness what modesty forbids. At all events we
> have never seen ladies in Europe taking such an undue interest in ceremonies
> like these, and we hope they will in future do as their mothers have done be-
> fore.[40]

The medical profession took a lively interest as well, drawing a distinction
between ritual and medical circumcision. By the 1880s, as more and more
Gentile physicians recommended and performed the operation as a neonatal
routine, they began to attack Jewish *berit milah* as primitive, unsanitary, and
dangerous.

Gentile doctors ridiculed those aspects of Jewish circumcision that recalled
blood ritual. B. Merrill Ricketts, a Cincinnati surgeon who kept fastidious
records of the hundreds of circumcisions he performed, quoted one of his fellow doctors who lamented the barbarism of "lower class" immigrants. "The
orthodox Jews have the habit of taking the organ into their mouth," he wrote
in disgust, "and sucking the blood after the operation has been performed."[41]
Stories of repulsive ritual practices, occasional reports of infection, gangrene,
tetanus in a Jewish infant who had been circumcised "in a very primitive
manner," and even reflex irritation *caused* by a clumsy operation stirred a chorus of opposition within the medical establishment. If it was to serve its purpose as a sanitary measure, the procedure should be performed "only by
medical men and in a surgical manner," a leading New York physician argued.
Poorly trained and ignorant of modern techniques, ritual circumcisers, he
wrote, occasionally infected infants with tuberculosis, syphilis, and other contagious microbes. In addition, Jews were thought to have a higher incidence
of hemophilia than other groups, and physicians assumed that a *mohel* who ac-
cidentally cut a hemophiliac's vein would be helpless to stop the bleeding. In

a scheme to regulate *mohels* out of existence, during the late 1880s doctors promoted a bill in the Ohio state legislature that would have banned ritual circumcision outright. Mainly because it violated the First Amendment, the measure never gained enough support to come to a vote. Despite repeated failures, the prospect of regulation—which would have shifted a good deal of business from unlicensed *mohels* to licensed Jewish physicians—was alluring to the medical profession. In New York, for example, a law proposed in 1900 aimed to strengthen the doctors' franchise by requiring that "at each and every operation, a duly registered and practicing physician shall be present, . . . shall superintend the operation, and shall be the responsible party."[42]

Outwardly, the intent of proposed regulations was to make the surgery safer, as one doctor urged, "by having the operation performed by a physician under antiseptic conditions." Godliness should not ignore cleanliness. All this talk of new laws, however, prompted one prominent Jewish doctor to quip that circumcision had become "the bête noire of our progressive Hebrew physicians imbued with the spirit of Listerism." Based on experience, he maintained that the *mohels*, far from spreading contagion, were fully abreast of modern techniques, their "armamentarium not complete without a bottle of carbolic and a strip of idioform gauze." If infection were a problem anywhere, he added, "we venture to say that in the best modern hospitals, where Listerism is carried out in a most rigorous way, sepsis occurs a hundredfold more than in the small crowded room where the Mohel is surgeon-in-chief." Could the explanation be, he asked, that unlike most physicians, the *mohel* was adept at cutting quickly and precisely, suppressing bleeding, and dressing the wound before infection had a chance to set in?[43]

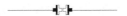

Over the decades, as squabbles about ritual circumcision faded away, the ethical issue of doing surgery on healthy patients was virtually ignored. Voices urging restraint were few and faint. One doctor in Brooklyn, N. M. Shaffer, lashed out at "indiscriminate circumcision" performed on infants and children who presented no symptoms of disease. Sir Herbert Snow, a prominent London cancer surgeon, published a pamphlet that received some attention in America, condemning "the barbarity of circumcision as a remedy for congenital abnormality." In 1894 an editorial in *Medical Record*, the New York Medical Society's official publication, ventured the opinion that "circumcision is a relic of barbarous and semicivilized times, before soap and water and sanitation had been preached. . . . In these days physicians should cease to preach or to impose upon their patients an unnecessary and irrational mutilation." Not that the writer was against sexual surgery altogether. "The rite which in these modern times might be substituted for the early religious ceremony of circumcision would, according to some, be resection of the spermatic cord of the vicious and defective classes, so they should cease to propagate their kind. Spermatorectomy will probably triumph over and replace circumcision, if anything does."[44] These were distinctly minority opinions. With the exception of that lone editorial, even the *Medical Record* was solidly in favor of circumcision, publishing dozens of papers extolling its benefits and promoting new surgical techniques.

No matter what physicians thought about circumcision, though, patients and parents made the ultimate decisions. In order to persuade healthy men to submit to genital surgery, or parents to make the decision on behalf of their male offspring, surgeons had to persuade them that it was a minor procedure, neither dangerous nor unduly painful. Two milestones, one theoretical and one technological, made this argument increasingly plausible.

First was the movement toward antisepsis, then asepsis, that followed germ theory. In Britain, Joseph Lister's pioneering work on antisepsis in surgery began in 1860. Using a combination of carbolic acid and heat to sterilize scalpels and clamps, he sharply reduced the rate of infections and postsurgical complications. Nonetheless, it took a generation for Lister's breakthrough, skeptically adopted by practicing surgeons, to produce aseptic surgery. By 1890, with the threat of hospital contagion dwindling, the medical world commenced an unprecedented boom in surgery. In 1800, according to medical historian Roy Porter, a leading London hospital might have done as many as 200 surgical procedures a year. A century later, the famous Mayo brothers and their assistants in Rochester, Minnesota, were performing 3,000 annually. More astonishing, by 1924 the Mayo Clinic logged 23,628 surgical cases. "The ambitious surgeon was beguiled into believing that all manner of diseases could be cured or checked," Porter writes, "by chloroforming the patient and plying the knife and the needle."[45]

New hospitals, typically outfitted with at least one freshly scrubbed surgical suite, sprouted up around the country like mushrooms. "To many surgeons," the historian Charles E. Rosenberg has remarked, the modern hospital "was beginning to seem the only ethical place to practice an increasingly demanding art." When Lewis Sayre performed his pioneering circumcisions for paralysis in the early 1870s, there were fewer than 200 hospitals in the United

States; forty years later there were more than 4,000, many of them for-profit ventures owned by physicians. This phenomenal increase in medical capacity naturally encouraged more operations of all kinds. Along the way, surgery came to seem increasingly routine and, for organs such as the tonsils and the prepuce, trivial.[46]

In immediate terms, asepsis meant less to patients than the other great breakthrough: effective anesthesia. Ether had entered the medical arena in the amphitheater of the Massachusetts General Hospital in 1846. Throughout the Civil War era, however, anesthetics—mainly ether, nitrous oxide, and chloroform—remained frighteningly unpredictable. Dosage was uncertain; techniques for administering anesthetic agents were slipshod. Children were particularly susceptible to complications, and the use of anesthesia in all but life-and-death cases remained controversial within the medical profession.

Not until the 1880s did medical scientists develop a variety of new drugs and safer procedures. A German ophthalmologist, Carl Koller, probably inspired by Sigmund Freud's work on the effects of cocaine, developed a cocaine solution that he used when operating on patients' eyes. Around the same time, American surgeon William Halsted published *Practical Comments on the Use and Abuse of Cocaine*, describing a hypodermic cocaine nerve block that could be used as a local anesthetic with little or no systemic effect. Lewis Sayre routinely chloroformed the patients he circumcised and reported no bad outcomes. For the many doctors who were leery of general anesthetics, however, cocaine administered locally appeared perfectly suited to circumcision.[47]

This innovation dramatically lowered the threshold for using the scalpel. C. Knox-Shaw spoke of giving a child "a few whiffs of chloroform, and at the same time twelve to fifteen minims of four per cent solution of cocaine . . . injected into the prepuce, about the level of the corona, in two or three places." Noting that over the years many of his patients had backed out of circumcision at the last minute "because I could not promise 'that it would not hurt,' " G. W. Overall said that by injecting cocaine, "now I can promise an operation where a child would not even know it until it was performed." He cited a case in which he had operated painlessly on a six-year-old boy "while he was discussing with his mother the kind of toys he would get for Christmas."[48]

Not every patient was so lucky. Evidence of pain and suffering of course is sparse. Physicians had little reason to document any distress that resulted from their actions. Patients and parents did not air private medical complaints in the press. The day when malpractice cases would become a common fixture at the plaintiffs' bar lay far off. Then as now, successful results were published, failures interred.

Still, in the shadows of journal articles and published comments one catches disturbing glimpses. "The text-books on surgery seem to imply that a circumcision is the simplest of procedures," Samuel Newman observed in the *Journal of the American Medical Association*. "The operation, however, is often troublesome." Inflammation, swelling, bleeding, and hematoma were fairly common postoperative complications. Every once in a while something worse happened: a staphylococcal infection, a severed nerve, an accidental amputation. Not that any of this should discourage doctors from operating, Newman said; all surgery carried some degree of risk. Jonathan Young Brown remarked that every surgeon who ever performed circumcision "has doubtless been struck with the fact, that almost invariably after the operation, the loose connective tissue lying between the remaining connective mucous and skin surfaces, become suddenly edematous, greatly swollen and occasionally almost tumefied. This condition delays or destroys union by the first intention, disfigures the part and renders the patient very uncomfortable." Safe as circumcision was, wrote Henry Simes, occasional problems were inevitable. In one unsettling incident, he had watched a colleague administer hydrochlorate of cocaine to a child, with terrible results. "Although the patient did not die, yet the effect was such that the operating surgeon then and there determined never to use the drug again for a similar operation." Worse, more than once, he recalled instances when "the surgeon, in operating, removed a portion of the glans."[49]

To help prevent surgical mishaps, medical journals published dozens of articles on new techniques and innovative medical devices. Advertisements extolled the merits of "Henry's phimosis forceps," guaranteed to render the procedure foolproof. Touting his patented "circumcision scissors" in two sizes, "a strong instrument for operating on adults, and a more delicate one for infants and children," Simon Baruch marveled at the proliferation of specially designed "clamps, forceps, and scissors" being sold to physicians. Only the imagination of surgeons limited the invention of new and ingenious methods. John W. Ross, proud purveyor of "Ross's Circumcision Ring," published "An Easy and Ready Method of Circumcision," instructing doctors on the ring's use. He contrived to insert "the glans penis up to the corona into the open mouth of a glass tube; tie a strong, small silk cord very tightly around the foreskin immediately in front of the flange of the tube; amputate the foreskin one-eighth of an inch in front of the constricting cord by a circular sweep of the knife; untie dressing; and keep the patient in bed, with penis elevated, for from twenty-four to forty-eight hours."[50]

Regardless of physicians' assurances that it was a minor procedure, circumcision seems to bear out the adage that the only minor surgery is that performed on someone else. Unless they suffered annoying symptoms, few men saw any reason to go under the knife. While no reliable data enable one to estimate the rate of medical circumcision at the turn of the century, the impression conveyed by dozens of articles in the contemporary medical literature is that the patients were mainly symptomatic middle- and upper-class children and teenagers. B. Merrill Ricketts kept the Cincinnati Medical Society apprised of his work in this field. In an 1894 paper, "The Last Fifty of a Series of Two Hundred Circumcisions," Ricketts listed twenty-nine indications for the operation.

LOCAL INDICATIONS		SYSTEMIC INDICATIONS
1. Hygienic	11. Cicatrices	1. Onanism
2. Phimosis	12. Inflammatory	2. Seminal emissions
3. Paraphimosis	thickening	3. Enuresis
4. Redundancy	13. Elephantiasis	
5. Adhesions	14. Nævus	4. Dysuria
6. Papillomata	15. Epithelioma	5. Retention
7. Eczema	16. Gangrene	6. General nervousness
(acute or chronic)	17. Tuberculosis	
8. Œdema	18. Preputial calculi	7. Impotence
9. Chancre	i) Hip-joint disease	8. Convulsions
10. Chancroid	ii) Hernia	9. Hystero-epilepsy

This list, especially the vague *Systemic Indications*, is so inclusive that most boys or men would have been likely to experience at least one of the symptoms. Whenever he had the chance, Ricketts performed surgeries for all these indications using "ordinary nickel-plated tailor's shears, with blades eight inches long and an inch wide, tapering down to a point," and professed that "there has been but one person of the two hundred upon whom I have operated who has regretted having had the operation of circumcision done." Ricketts was at the forefront; before the turn of the century, physicians could not take popular acceptance for granted. When they recommended circumcision, they expected dubiousness, and so polished their arguments to overcome it.[51]

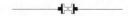

The ultimate popularity of circumcision depended not on convincing normal men to undergo the ordeal of surgery, but on targeting a group of patients who could not object. From the mid-1880s onward, physicians and at their behest, parents, came to suppose that the theory and practice of circumcision applied most ideally to infants. When performed on babies, a New York doctor maintained, "circumcision is no more of an operation than vaccination." And as Jews had long since discovered, babies tolerated it without requiring chloroform or cocaine. "Infants only a few years old may be held down by two assistants and the operation done without any anesthetic," Samuel Newman advised. For his own part, Newman preferred to bind his young patients "to a board after the Indian fashion of strapping the papoose . . . to hold the child firmly in place until the operation is ended."[52]

If one acknowledged the many benefits claimed for circumcision—if parents accepted the vaccination analogy—it made sense to operate as early as possible, before diseases and nasty habits had a chance to take hold.[53]

The 1880s represent a turning point in children's medicine. Earlier, in medical terms, children were regarded simply as little people, not a separate class of patients. After public health agencies began to document shocking rates of infant mortality, however—especially in urban areas—the medical profession organized to combat childhood diseases. In 1880, under President Lewis Sayre's aegis, the AMA instituted a new section of pediatric medicine. Four years later, the first specialist journal devoted to children's medicine appeared, the *Archives of Pediatrics*; and in 1887, the American Pediatric Society held its first meeting.

These organizational shifts exemplified a new view of the proper relationship between organized medicine and children. Aptly, the pediatric movement's guiding light was Abraham Jacobi, president of the New York Medical Society and a tireless crusader. The hallmark of Jacobi's pediatric medicine was reassessment of all facets of children's minds and bodies, and entrance by physicians into areas formerly the private domain of families. Doubtless the best-known example of pediatric activism was the baby feeding controversy. Doctors rallied to save American babies from mothers' milk, which they declared unsafe. Testing their growing cultural authority, pediatricians concocted and pushed an assortment of infant formulas and special bottles designed to replace breast-feeding.[54] What sparked the infant formula movement were hospital data showing that diarrheal disorders constituted a leading cause of infant mortality, responsible for as many as one in four deaths.

Searching for ways to prevent gastrointestinal illness, pediatric specialists recommended not only feeding babies "pure" formulas, but also removing the foreskins of newborn boys. Eliminating a prime source of irritation from the nervous system—namely, the prepuce—seemed sure to aid a baby's digestion, thereby improving his chances for survival. J. A. Hofheimer, in a widely cited article, reported success in using circumcision to cure both fecal incontinence and constipation. Encouraged by his results, he recommended operating at once, before symptoms had a chance to appear. "An early operation," he wrote, "will relieve the child of a great source of irritation, and indirectly improve nutrition; changing a fretful, puny baby into a thriving, happy infant." Putting this advice to a test in the case of an incontinent, dehydrated child, Doctor H. L. Rosenberry confessed that he had no idea why it worked, but the patient soon became healthy and robust. "I am at a loss to explain the process," he said somewhat apologetically, "but simply relate it as a fact."[55]

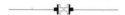

As an omnibus procedure, effective against dozens of widely feared yet poorly understood disorders, circumcision was inevitably enlisted in the late-Victorian war on masturbation. Anglo-American culture was notoriously ill at ease with human sexuality. Indeed, medical thought in the late nineteenth century contained one central principle about male sexuality. The governing assumption was that man's sexual impulse was by nature aggressive, dangerous, destructive, and indeed the most subversive of human appetites. Just how imperfectly the bonds of work, culture, and society held male lust in check was apparent in the cities, with their rising rates of illegitimate births and epidemics of venereal disease.

The censorious, neo-Puritan Comstock Act of 1873 expressed the anxiety about sex that simmered within the middle and upper classes. For these groups, manifestations of infant and child sexuality were especially disturbing, at odds with their idealized image of children's natural purity. In ages past, children's tendency to play with their genitals had provoked little serious concern; but amidst a general shift in sexual attitudes during the middle decades of the nineteenth century, popular views of masturbation darkened. Since the Enlightenment, doctors in Western Europe and America had occasionally identified masturbation as a cause of illnesses. In the course of the nineteenth century it was linked to madness, idiocy, epilepsy, and, as the idea of reflex irritation gained currency, a multitude of other conditions, all bad. "Let it be known that pulmonary consumption, whose horrible ravages in Europe ought to give alarm to all governments, has drawn from this very source its fatal power," proclaimed popular New York physician and author Joseph W. Howe. If tuberculosis were not enough, "the most serious forms of disorder attributable to this cause are *spinal paralysis, locomotor-ataxia,* and *convulsions*," declared a physician at Virginia's South-Western Asylum. "Besides these, masturbation, does occasionally, induce an intractable form of insanity." This was so-called masturbatory insanity, a label many American and British physicians attached to psychotic illnesses they could not otherwise classify.[56]

Judaism, and later Catholicism, had long insisted that masturbation, because it spent a precious resource God intended purely for marriage and procreation, was a terrible sin. By squandering his "seed," the masturbator was guilty of a crime as serious as abortion or even, in the opinion of some commentators, murder. The Talmud harshly condemned the practice. And the *Zohar*, an influential commentary within the mystical Jewish tradition, condemned masturbation as "a sin more serious than all the sins of the Torah." To avoid temptation, according to Jewish law, one should take pains to avoid sexual arousal. The penis should not be touched: "the unmarried man never, and the married man only in connection with urination." It was said that when Orthodox Jews trained their young sons to urinate, they admonished them, "Without hands! Better a bad aim than a bad habit."[57]

Implausible as it sounds, leading Jewish physicians maintained that circumcision served to immunize Jewish boys and men against the bad habit of masturbation. During the spring of 1860, a series of articles published in Britain's leading medical journal, *The Lancet*, reported that masturbation and bed-wetting were comparatively rare in Jewish communities. Several years later, on the other side of the Atlantic, while Lewis Sayre was circumcising boys for paralysis and epilepsy, Abraham Jacobi and M. J. Moses (one the organizer of the American Pediatric Society, the other head of the New York State Medical Society, and president of the Association of American Physicians), crusaded against the foreskin as the primary cause of masturbation. "As an Israelite, I desire to ventilate the subject, and, as a physician, have chosen the medium of a medical journal, that I may not be trammeled in my expressions, as I necessarily would be were I confined to the pages of an ordinary paper," wrote Moses. "I refer to masturbation as one of the effects of a long prepuce; not that this vice is entirely absent in those who have undergone circumcision, though I never saw an instance in a Jewish child of very tender years, except as the result of association with children whose covered glans have naturally impelled them to the habit."[58]

Righteous people have always sought to avoid sin. Yet the medical theory that masturbation provoked disease presented a more present threat. Fittingly in the era of Darwin, nature's laws and medical science joined God as punishers of transgression. Athol A. W. Johnson advised doctors to perform the procedure without chloroform "so that the pain experienced may be associated with the habit we wish to eradicate." In America, this idea was promoted by John Harvey Kellogg, a surgeon at the Battle Creek Sanitarium who gained fame for his obsession with dietary fiber and bowel disorders. Pronouncing it "almost always successful in small boys," Kellogg recommended performing circumcision "without administering an anesthetic, as the pain attending the operation will have a salutary effect upon the mind, especially if connected with the idea of punishment." The sadistic theme of inflicting a just measure of pain (for the patient's own good) forms a common thread in the medical literature around the turn of the century. "I performed an orificial operation," wrote one surgeon with barely concealed delight. Having become addicted to "the secret vice practiced among boys," the young patient "needed the rightful punishment of cutting pains after his illicit pleasures."[59]

Using circumcision as a combination of punishment and prevention was probably not uncommon. A. E. Housman (1869–1936), the distinguished British poet and scholar, seems to have suffered enduring anguish from the circumcision his father forced on him and his brothers when he was fourteen. Houseman suffered permanent trauma, and some scholars have identified the event as the source of the poet's sexual preoccupation with humiliation, mutilation, and violent death.[60]

Late-nineteenth-century physicians battled masturbation with the same unstinting zeal their descendants would employ in the war against illegal drugs. As for solid evidence that masturbation caused disease—a notion that gained almost universal acceptance inside and outside the medical profession—this came mainly from physicians' experience with mentally ill patients. "There can be no doubt of [masturbation's] injurious effects," declared a Philadelphia doctor with the peculiar name of Angel Money, "and of the proneness to practice it on the part of children with defective brains." In addition to circumcision, he advised his colleagues "to make the genitals so sore by blistering fluids that pain results from attempts to rub the parts."[61]

It was unnerving, an asylum doctor wrote, to see the hands of the feebleminded "instinctively drawn to those parts." Based on nothing more than observations like this, he and many others decided that masturbation caused lunacy. Of course, the mechanism of cause and effect remained cryptic. Since evidently there were lots of chronic masturbators whose minds continued to function quite normally, Remondino noted, "it may be a question as to whether the feeble-mindedness be not a reflex condition from this excessive morbid irritability of the sexual organs." Other commentators, pediatricians prominently among them, warned parents that masturbation was learned in infancy and that the foreskin was chiefly to blame. "The fact that children under two years of age can and frequently do contract the habit of masturbation is a revelation to many physicians," declared J. P. Webster in a paper he read to the Ohio Pediatric Society. He went on to profile a typical masturbator: a three-year-old boy who was "small, had a scowl on his face, looked wearied and bloated; he was nervous and fretful, a poor eater and a very poor sleeper." The sickly child had developed his habit before he was a year old, according to Webster, evidently "due in the first place to the condition of the prepuce."[62]

When in 1896 a popular book, *All About Baby*, advised mothers that circumcision of baby boys was "advisable in most cases," it recommended the operation mainly for preventing "the vile habit of masturbation." L. Emmett Holt, professor at the College of Physicians and Surgeons in Philadelphia, and a distinguished expert on pediatric medicine, told his fellow physicians that "adherent prepuce . . . is so constantly present that it can hardly be called a malformation. It is, however, a condition needing attention in every male infant." The perils of neglect, he said, included "priapism, masturbation, insomnia, night terrors, etc.," and for that matter, "most of the functional nervous diseases of childhood." Peter Remondino, for his part, was certain that "circumcised boys may, in individual cases . . . be found to practice onanism, but in general the practice can be asserted as being very rare among the children of circumcised races . . . neither in infancy are they as liable to priapism during sleep as those that are uncircumcised."[63]

One physician who described successfully circumcising an infant to cure urinary tract lithuria also remembered having detected similar "oxalic acid deposits in the urine of masturbators, and *offspring-shunning husbands*, who practice onanism." In his mind, this observation not only reconfirmed the theory that masturbation was connected with neurasthenic disease but more important, implied that the habit itself was a response to an anatomical disorder. In the view of many practitioners, masturbation was simply an intermediate link in a chain of cause-and-effect that originated in the foreskin.[64]

Odd as it may seem for an operation supposed to suppress masturbation, Remondino and others also endorsed circumcision as protection against impotence. A syndrome often untraceable to any specific cause, impotence fit into the theoretical framework that supported circumcision. Possibly the foreskin frayed the nerves by its presence; possibly it harbored germs that weakened the penis; or perhaps, as one surgical textbook described phimosis, "the prepuce gets behind the corona glandis, threatening the strangulation of the organ." However it happened, the prepuce threatened healthy sexuality. "Sexual relations are much more to man or woman than is generally acknowledged," Remondino declared, and freeing the male organ from "a constricting, unnatural band" would surely enhance sexual performance and pleasure. In uncircumcised men, an elongated, contracted prepuce could induce sterility. "Before the wife is censured, in every case where the marriage is unfruitful, the husband should submit to an examination," he admonished his profession. "If an abnormal condition of the prepuce is found, circumcision should be advised and results awaited."[65]

Presaging arguments made by circumcision opponents several decades later, an English surgeon named Jonathan Hutchinson conceded that removing the foreskin in all likelihood did rob a man of tactility. But this was not a bad thing. For if the only physiological benefit of the prepuce "is that of maintaining the penis in a condition susceptible to more acute sensation than would otherwise exist," Hutchinson wrote, "it may increase the pleasure of coition and the impulse to it." Fortunately, though, thanks to circumcision, "these are advantages which in the present state of society can well be spared." By rendering the penis less sensitive, circumcision enhanced sexual self-control, he continued, something for which "one should be thankful." E. Harding Freeland, arguing for circumcision in the pages of the *Lancet*, shared this opinion. "Whatever may have been the case in days gone by," he declared in 1900, "sensuality in our time needs neither whip nor spur, but would be all the better for a little more judicious use of curb and bearing-rein."[66]

The cumulative weight of expert opinion inevitably changed physician behavior. In the early years of the twentieth century, circumcision steadily became a standard practice for well-trained doctors. Although hospitals and doctors seldom kept statistics, on the eve of World War I a physician making a case for "Universal Circumcision as a Sanitary Measure" in the *Journal of the American Medical Association* estimated the number of children who had undergone the procedure in the "millions." Surveying medical opinion all around America, and in Britain as well, he felt confident that "the vast preponderance of modern scientific opinion on the subject is strongly in favor of circumcision as a sanitary measure and as a prophylactic against infection with venereal disease." What few scruples remained were not against removing the foreskin, he added, "but against those persons who fail to do it properly." Articles published throughout the 1920s support this view. Whether or not to circumcise was hardly at issue. All that remained was to ensure the best technique.[67]

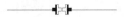

Perfecting surgical technique was important to avoid mishaps and also to create an attractive result. Aesthetics mattered, for circumcision was becoming a mark of social distinction. In the early years of the twentieth century, it was the emerging social meaning of the operation that enshrined it in popular culture where it would flourish long after the theories that originally inspired it were forgotten.

Except for a few experiments Lewis Sayre and others carried out on boys in state mental institutions, medical circumcision in its early phase was reserved mainly for the carriage trade: better-off patients who could afford it. Consequently, medical men grew accustomed to thinking of the procedure in class terms. Advising his readers that the earliest known circumcisions were the prerogative of the priest caste of ancient Egypt, Peter Remondino drew an analogy between ancient and modern practice. Though few people realized it, he said, America was home to a group of spiritual descendants of the Egyptian priests, "a class which also observe circumcision as a hygienic precaution, where, from my personal observation, I have found that circumcision is thoroughly practiced in every male member of many of the families of the class—this being the physician class." Whether as a result of their medical training or of seeing at first hand "the many dangers and disadvantages that follow the uncircumcised," he said, American physicians were quietly subjecting themselves to the procedure. Having done so, "instead of being dissatisfied, they have extended the advantages they have themselves received, by having those in their charge likewise operated upon." As Remondino saw it, circumcision proliferated *sotto voce* as a guild secret for a privileged few, the mark of a modern, scientific elite.[68]

Learning of its advantages in the privacy of their physicians' offices, Americans found circumcision appealing not merely on medical grounds, but also for its connotations of science, health, and cleanliness—newly important class distinctions. Around the turn of the century, immigrants were surging in from southern and Eastern Europe, inundating the industrial centers in the Northeast and Midwest, drastically changing the demography of American cities.

Between 1890 and 1914, 17 million foreigners arrived. This human influx confronted old-stock Americans with a crisis of cultural identity. Faced with millions of foreigners, living in the sort of urban poverty more typical of the industrial centers of the Old World, the guardians of American purity scorned the new arrivals as racially inferior. They were Europe's "wretched refuse of your teeming shore" according to Emma Lazarus's memorable inscription on the base of the Statue of Liberty. Congress rushed to pass anti-immigration legislation, politicians and the popular press likened the new immigrants to a human wave of filth and pollution, a grave threat to America's body politic. Lurid rhetoric and genuine apprehension about assimilating disparate groups fueled a national obsession with contamination and thus with sanitation. New York's Ellis Island, the point of entry for millions, was celebrated for cleanliness; its showers were equipped to handle 8,000 immigrants a day.

This dread of filth was a rich cultural stew. Beliefs about pollution and contamination—whether from masturbation, asbestos, or plutonium—are loaded with symbolism. A culture's rules for distinguishing the clean from the unclean, as anthropologist Mary Douglas has shown in her study *Purity and Danger*, contain "analogies for expressing a general view of the social order." Clean and dirty are powerful expressions of hierarchy and measures of social distance.[69]

Medical circumcision thus assumed a special role in the fin-de-siècle search for rank and social order. It signified precisely that aversion to dirt—and not just dirt, but vulgarity, nasty habits, and diseases—that symbolically set one on a higher plane. Undoubtedly this was the enduring core of its appeal to ordinary people. It was during these decades that the idea of "normal" first acquired its cultural force. The philosopher Ian Hacking suggests that normality "displaced the Enlightenment idea of human nature as an organizing concept."[70] Out of the complicated social milieu at the turn of the twentieth century—when eugenics was another attractive public health measure—grew an ideal of the normal healthy body: nature's product improved by modern surgery. Ultimately, the surgically altered state was deemed normal.

With each passing year, maternity care and childbirth for the middle and upper classes was changing from a domestic event managed by midwives, relatives, and friends into a medical event managed by physicians. Since midwives rarely performed circumcisions, for Gentiles having one's foreskin removed became a sign of having been delivered by a physician. Doctors suggested it to parents immediately after the birth of a son. Circumcision, they professed, was based on state-of-the-art medical knowledge. Done in the germ-free confines of the hospital, the operation itself was simple and eminently safe, and it reduced the infant's risk from the deadly diseases of childhood. Parents usually acquiesced. And so circumcision became a token of the medicalization of childbirth, literally a symbol of the rising authority of the medical profession over the laity.[71]

On a more mundane level, circumcision promised to spare parents the ordeal of someday having to deal with masturbation. It meant that a boy's parents had given him every chance, providing him with proper medical care from the beginning. It thus became a responsibility for sensible parents. Frank G. Lydston bluntly emphasized this point in his popular 1912 treatise on social hygiene when he wrote, *"parents who do not have an early circumcision performed on their boys are almost criminally negligent."*[72]

So it came about that the foreskin, viewed as dangerous by the medical profession, commonly came to indicate ignorance, neglect, and poverty. As white middle-class Gentiles adopted circumcision, those left behind were recent immigrants, people of color, the poor, and others at the margins of respectable society. These were the groups imagined to have filthy, malodorous bodies: people who lacked culture, manners, intelligence, and, in a word, civilization.[73]

FIVE

The Fabric of the Foreskin

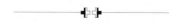

There is no structure in the body that can be described as simple.

—*Sherwin B. Nuland,* The Wisdom of the Body *(1997)*

MEDICAL SUPPORT FOR ROUTINE CIRCUMCISION HAS RESTED ON A PRESUMPTION that the foreskin is trivial, as one physician quipped, just a few millimeters of skin. Few doctors would as a matter of course remove tissue covering the glans penis if they believed it served a biological purpose. Yet books and articles written about the male reproductive organs offer amazingly little in the way of detailed nuts-and-bolts analysis. Since the nineteenth century, scientists have realized that organs are complex systems and that one of the supreme challenges of anatomy is to discover the functional coordination between various components of the body. Historically, this process of understanding was limited to gross anatomical observation, first with the naked eye, then assisted by increasingly powerful microscopes. Recently, powerful imaging technologies have made it possible to focus on the interaction of molecules. As our understanding of the body deepens, even a few millimeters of skin may demonstrate the wisdom of the body.

The trivialization of the prepuce is of fairly recent vintage, produced by circumcision advocates toward the end of the nineteenth century. Throughout Western history, most anatomists considered the prepuce not merely a bit of excess tissue but an essential part of the sexual organ itself.

The classic paradigm for medical thinking about the foreskin was what historian Thomas Laqueur calls "the one-sex model." Articulated by Aristotle and generally accepted by physicians and educated laymen alike for two thousand years, this model represented male and female genitalia as mirror images of each other. Early cartographers of human anatomy perceived woman as man inverted: "the uterus was the female scrotum, the ovaries were testicles, the vulva was a foreskin, and *the vagina was a penis*." Galen, the second-century anatomical sage, succinctly explained the theory to his students. "Turn outward the woman's, turn inward, so to speak, and fold double the man's [genital organs]" he instructed, "and you will find them the same in both in every respect." Describing the female sex organs, Galen's contemporary, Soranus, whose observations set a standard for gynecological anatomy that would endure through the Renaissance, noted, "The inner part of the vagina grows around the neck of the uterus like the prepuce in the male around the glans." To Soranus and his followers, the prepuce was an integral structure of genitalia, male and female. In the words of Renaissance anatomist Gabriello Fallopio, "All parts that are in men are present in women."[1]

The analogy stuck. In the mid-sixteenth century, Charles Estienne, distinguished anatomist to Francis I, published a book based on his many dissections. Of genitalia, he wrote, "Whatever one sees in women as a kind of opening in the vaginal orifice, one finds the same in the foreskin of the male privy parts, a sort of hollowed-out protuberance. The only difference between the two is that in woman the hollowness is far greater than in man." Important as gross anatomy was to understanding how the body works, it proved impossible for anatomists to discard the legends and traditions embedded in their training. Before the sixteenth century, for example, it was common knowledge that a male carried one fewer rib than a female, owing to God's first surgery on Adam, as described in the Book of Genesis.[2]

During the Renaissance, Italian anatomists such as Niccolo Massa and Alessandro Benedetti, systematically mapping the body, naturally included the foreskin. "The skin covering the penis is remarkable for its thinness, its dark colour, and its looseness of connexion with the fascial sheath of the organ," reads a characteristic description. "At the neck of the penis, it is folded upon itself to form the prepuce or foreskin, which covers the glans for a variable distance."[3]

Jacopo Berengario da Carpi, the first scholar to publish an illustrated anatomical text, described the foreskin as "a certain soft skin" surrounding the glans, "obedient to reversion [pulling back] at any rubbing. This prepuce in the lower part in the middle only along its length is attached to the larger part of the glans by a certain pellicular member vulgarly called 'the little thread'" (*il filello*). What functions did the male foreskin perform? Berengario thought that its purposes were both erogenous, "to furnish some delight in coitus," and protective, "to guard the glans from external harm." The male organ was just as sensitive as the female, but because it hung outside the body it was especially vulnerable, "apt to dry out and close up." Berengario considered Jewish circumcision, because it cut away this needed layer of protection, to be "operating against the intent of nature." Expanding on Aristotle's mirroring of male and female genitalia, he also observed that the "neck of the womb" is guarded by the labia just as "the skin of the prepuce guards the penis." Similarly, in the female body, "at the end of the cervix little skins are added at the sides; these are called prepuces." Berengario even used the same word (*nymphae*) to describe the labia majora, labia minora, and the male foreskin.[4]

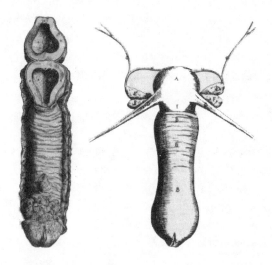

On the left is Vesalius's rendering of the vagina from *De humani corporis fabrica* (1543); on the right is the vagina and uterus from Vidus Vidius, *De anatome corporis humani* (1611). Both images represent the vagina as a penislike organ.

Fallopio, whose virtuoso dissections described in *Observationes Anatomicae* (1565) enabled him to detail fine structures from the optical nerves to the eponymous fallopian tubes, pushed the analogy a step further. The prepuce played a role not merely in sexual pleasure, he postulated, but in procreation, because human conception depended on both sexual partners reaching orgasm. Failing that, no vital seed would be produced. The foreskin supplied the penis with "natural lubricity," heightening erotic sensation. And "when the pleasure is greater," he wrote, "the woman emits seed and suitable material for the formation of the foetus."[5]

Throughout the sixteenth and seventeenth centuries, from the celebrated public dissections in Bologna to the operating theaters of London, anatomical learning multiplied—and the foreskin was described as part of the penis. If it became diseased, physicians and surgeons endeavored to outline the best courses of treatment. The immensely learned and influential French surgeon Abroise Paré wrote of phimosis and paraphimosis, advising when circumcision was indicated to cure these disorders and describing the best methods of operation. Believing there was value in retaining the prepuce, he described a procedure to restore the foreskin of a man who had lost his.[6] William Harvey, the eminent English physician who first described blood circulation, thought the prepuce enhanced erotic sensation. "The circumcised are affected with less pleasure in coitus," he wrote, "because the membrane is thickened and sensation blunted." Addressing the question of why people in antiquity had originated the operation, he cojectured that it had been invented by tribes in hot climates to prevent leprosy, a disease he identified with dirt and filth.[7]

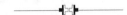

It remained for the nineteenth century, blending reflex neurosis theory, half-formed notions of Darwinian evolution, and an exaggerated dread of masturbation, to recast the foreskin as a hazard. Even though this was a period of vigorous anatomical research, however, the medical reappraisal of the foreskin was not based on new insight into its structure and function. Quite the opposite. Case reports, clinical series, and anecdotes, which constituted most of the medical literature about circumcision and the foreskin between 1870 and 1920, produced a collective image rife with myths and misconceptions. Students in leading medical schools such as Johns Hopkins in Baltimore were taught that the prepuce was tantamount to a minor birth defect and was a source of future problems, which they as physicians should quickly correct soon after a boy was born. To prevent phimosis before it started, interns were trained to retract an infant's or young child's foreskin by applying as much force as necessary. Tissue adhesion and the bleeding caused by forcible retraction were considered proof of incipient foreskin problems and thus were indications for circumcision.[8]

All bodily organs present a wide range of variation. What is considered normal—in size, shape, color, and other attributes—is the median range of a bell curve. In the clinic, normal is generally a standard in the eye of the physician. Indeed, the ability to distinguish what is normal (and best left alone) from what is disordered (and requires treatment) has always been central to the art of medicine. Unfortunately, medical literature from the early decades of the twentieth century shows that the Anglo-American medical community shared

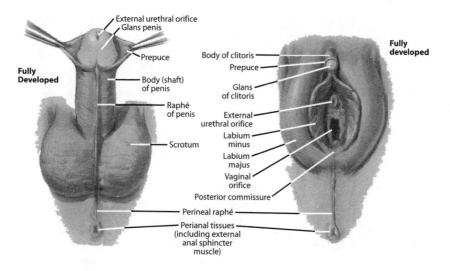

Male and female external genitalia. From Frank H. Netter, M.D., *Atlas of Human Anatomy* (1989); reproduced by permission of Novartis Medical Education..

faulty assumptions about what the developing penis should look like and how the foreskin should function.

Voices urging a more considered approach fell on deaf ears. In 1916, Geoffrey Jefferson, a hospital pathologist in British Columbia, took time to dissect, stain, and examine ten prepuces under his microscope. He expected to observe simple flaps of skin. Writing up his findings, however, he professed astonishment at the amount of muscle tissue in his specimens and the complex connections of the peripenic muscle within the muscular structure of the penis. This laboratory research, along with his experience in the clinic, led him to conclude that the foreskin was unusually dynamic, both in muscular activity and in long-term development from infancy to maturity. "It is inconceivable that children are born with actual deformities in this region as often as the statistics would lead an observer to suppose," Jefferson wrote. What his profession regularly diagnosed as "redundancy of the foreskin," he noted, "is not only common but normal; the skin awaits the development of the *corpora cavernosa* and *spongiosum* which will occur at puberty." By the same token, he was suspicious of the diagnosis of phimosis in a neonate because in a boy's early years "adhesion between the prepuce and the glans is not an absolute abnormality, nor one which time cannot correct."[9]

Through the 1940s, anatomists occasionally published papers dealing with the prepuce. They showed that, like the rest of the penis, it developed a profuse network of capillaries, blood vessels, and nerves. Logically this made it a significant source of sensation, though no one drew this inference.[10] Nevertheless, it was not until midcentury that anyone reconsidered the prepuce in fuller perspective—and in the process, directly assaulted conventional wisdom.

In December 1949, Douglas Gairdner, a respected English pediatrician affiliated with the United Cambridge Hospitals, published a provocative paper in the *British Medical Journal* titled "The Fate of the Foreskin: A Study of Circumcision." Gairdner began by saying that he found it curious that one of his country's most common operations had received so little rigorous attention. Sensibly, he reasoned that "in order to decide whether a child's foreskin should be ablated the normal anatomy and function of the structure at different ages should be understood; the danger of conserving the foreskin must then be weighed against the hazards of the operation, the mortality and after-effects of which must be known." Despite the tens of thousands of circumcisions performed annually, he continued, nobody had undertaken a systematic analysis. In consequence, data on which to decide the question were insufficient.[11]

Gairdner's critique, though revolutionary, did not come out of the blue. In the wake of World War II, Britain had established a compulsory, cradle-to-grave medical insurance program. As they drew up lists of what medical procedures would be covered under the new scheme, architects of the new government-funded National Health Service (NHS) were forced explicitly to confront questions about costs and benefits. How much taxpayer money should be allocated to doctors and hospitals? Where should one draw the line between an essential service and one that, even though a patient might desire it and a doctor might be willing to perform it, was not medically necessary? Such issues were novel and complex, yet physicians and laypeople alike knew they must be confronted if the NHS program was to work within a limited budget.

During the war, circumcision already had been curtailed to conserve medical resources. In peacetime, doctors reverted to their old ways. With the British economy in serious recession during the late 1940s, however, one essential function of the NHS was to rein in the medical economy by rationing medical services. Rationing implied a selective allocation of money. Theoretically, Gairdner believed, if routine circumcision proved unnecessary, Britain could shift resources to other more valuable interventions.

So he started at the beginning, with a lesson in the anatomy and development of the normal prepuce. Eight weeks after conception, he wrote, a male fetus normally begins to develop "a ring of thickened epidermis" that grows, over the next eight weeks, to the tip of the glans penis. In the early stages, the skin tissue of the prepuce is not differentiated from the epidermis covering the glans, "both consisting of squamous epithelium." With time, these squamous cells form patterns of whorls. The cells at the center of the whorls die, creating a series of tiny empty pockets. Gradually these pockets expand and connect with each other, opening larger and larger spaces between the prepuce and the glans until, at some point (usually a considerable time after the child is born) "a continuous preputial space is formed." Gairdner emphasized that individuals developed at vastly different rates. Illustrations of sections of the penis in three full-term newborn boys showed a wide range, from the prepuce being completely separated from the glans at one extreme to the process of foreskin separation not even having begun at the other.[12]

Gairdner knew that based on what they had learned in textbooks and their experience with older male patients, most doctors expected the prepuce and glans penis to be separate structures from birth. Since the late nineteenth century, the term *adherent prepuce* (meaning that some "adhesion" impeded the foreskin from being pulled back off the glans penis) had been an accepted indication for circumcision, first in men, then in boys, and finally in babies. In 1933, a respected American authority on neonatal anatomy at Jefferson Medical College, Glenn Deibert, advised physicians that while typically incomplete at birth, "separation is sufficient at the 10-day state to allow mechanical retraction without danger of a tear." Not unreasonably, doctors assumed that if infants' foreskins adhered to the glans it was evidence of a problem.[13]

Such thinking, Gairdner made clear, ignored normal developmental variation. Based on a sample of 300 patients—100 newborns and 200 boys up to the age of five—he found that just 4 percent were born with a fully retractable foreskin; 54 percent had some limited measure of retractability; and in 42 percent the prepuce was so firmly attached that even the tip of the glans could not be uncovered. It loosened as the boys grew older. Even at 6 months, though, the foreskin was nonretractable in four out of every five boys. By the first birthday, the group divided about evenly. Subsequently, they continued to develop, albeit at different rates: "By 2 years about 20% and by 3 years about 10% of boys still have a non-retractable prepuce." With a three-year-old, wrote Gairdner, if minor adhesion presented a problem, it was easy enough insert a

probe between the glans penis and foreskin gently to ease apart the attached
tissues. In a sample of fifty-four boys referred to the United Cambridge Hospitals for circumcision, most of them diagnosed with phimosis, Gairdner observed that all but one were successfully treated with the probe. In the single
exception, an infant five months old, "the manoeuvre failed because preputial
separation had not advanced far enough to enable manipulation to complete
the process." As far as he was concerned it was foolish to try to force retraction in a child so young, since in most cases this would mean tearing apart "as
yet incompletely separated surfaces." Beyond the pain it caused, forced retraction often induced bleeding and opened fresh channels for infection. Too often ignorance produced an iatrogenic disease—a disorder caused not by
nature, but by the meddling of a well-intentioned doctor.[14]

Forcible retraction has remained a problem in the clinic. Canadian pediatric
specialists who studied the matter in 1996 observed that "in general, there is inadequate recognition of the long period before the natural separation of the
prepuce and glans is complete." They noted that papers in medical journals
continued to refer to "adhesions" in toddlers, as though their foreskins should
have been fully retractable. In England and America, many practitioners assumed that an unretractable foreskin means phimosis, leading to referrals for
circumcision to correct the condition. Even in Japan, where circumcision was
little known before World War II, modern American medicine influenced doctors to diagnose preputial unretractability as a medical problem. In 1996, a team
of pediatric researchers at Akita's Fujiwara Hospital evaluated 603 Japanese boys
from newborns to fifteen-year-olds only to conclude, "incomplete separation
of the prepuce is common and normal in neonates and infants, and preputial
separation progresses until adolescence." They expressed hope that their findings would reduce Japan's increasing rate of unnecessary circumcisions.[15]

Gairdner also looked at an older group of 200 uncircumcised boys between the ages of five and thirteen years old. About one in five had some
problem retracting the prepuce. This included 6 percent of the cohort who
could not retract it at all. Upon examination Gairdner discovered that in most
cases the restriction was nothing more than "the persistence of a few strands
of tissue between prepuce and glans." These could be treated simply and con-
servatively using the probe technique. He considered this desirable, especially
after the age of five or so, because unless they could easily pull back the prepuce to wash themselves, older boys secreted smegma that was malodorous
and, Gairdner feared, a potential risk factor for cancer.[16]

Responding to the supposition "that the prepuce is a vestigial structure devoid of function," Gairdner maintained that before a baby was toilet trained,

while he was in diapers the foreskin offered the sensitive skin of the glans some protection from irritating contact with urine and feces. Skin eruptions on the glans known as "metal ulcer," he noted, rarely occurred in uncircumcised children, and then only in instances "when the prepuce happens to be unusually lax and the glans constantly exposed." He did not venture any opinions about how the prepuce might enhance sexual response, except to comment dryly "that whenever the subject has been broached in male company, those still in possession of their foreskin have been forward in their insistence that any differences which may exist in such matters operate emphatically to their own advantage."[17]

When one considers the circumcision controversy that erupted in America in the 1970s, it seems surprising that Gairdner's paper and the subsequent decision by the NHS not to cover circumcision except for diagnosed disease caused so little stir. Perhaps this was because Gairdner went with the economic grain, rationalizing medicine and saving money in a time of scarcity.

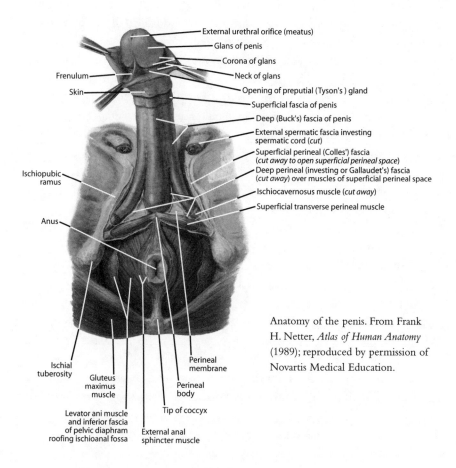

Anatomy of the penis. From Frank H. Netter, *Atlas of Human Anatomy* (1989); reproduced by permission of Novartis Medical Education.

In America, where a system of private insurance left individual doctors to determine what was medically appropriate, Gairdner was all but ignored. Circumcision was standard practice, its legitimacy bolstered by the American military experience. Physicians in the armed forces strongly believed that the foreskin was a risk factor for venereal diseases—a source of intense paranoia during the war—and encouraged uncircumcised recruits to undergo the operation. Impressed by the fact that most officers and soldiers from affluent families were circumcised, thousands of enlisted soldiers and sailors signed up for circumcisions in military hospitals before returning to civilian life.

Meanwhile, the phenomenal postwar boom in medical research, funded by bountiful increases in government support for agencies such as the National Institutes of Health, ensured that every facet of human anatomy and physiology would come under new scrutiny.

Surveying the state of knowledge in the late 1950s, an anatomical researcher commented on the "many diverse judgments" his predecessors had made about the prepuce, and the paucity of data to support any of them. Over the years, the foreskin becomes comparatively shorter: "the glans remains completely covered in only 45 percent of men, partially covered in 32 percent and is completely uncovered (auto-circumcision) in 23 percent." There is racial variation: the foreskin is typically longer in Africans, shorter in Chinese and Japanese.[18] One contribution was to detail "the deep and superficial network of nerve fibres in the dermis" of the prepuce. The prepuce, wrote R. K. Winkelmann, qualified as an erogenous zone, whose "anatomy favors acute perception." Unlike most of the body's skin, on close examination the prepuce displayed a nerve network quite similar to that of the glans. The main feature was a dense spiraling of Vater-Pacini corpuscles, clusters of fine-tuned nerve endings associated with exquisite sensation.[19]

American doctors were so accustomed to thinking of the foreskin as worthless and of those who retained it as dirty that mainstream journals entertained no real criticism of circumcision until the 1960s. In 1970, Captain E. Noel Preston, a staff pediatrician at California's Vandenberg Air Force Base, published a sober critique of standard practice under the tongue-in-cheek title "Whither the Foreskin?" Citing Gairdner's earlier work, he told the membership of the American Medical Association that in his experience, the conditions they were used to thinking of as disorders of the prepuce were for the most part normal and unthreatening. A common reason for excising the foreskin was to prevent phimosis. But, he said, "actually the presence of phimosis cannot be determined at birth because histologically the prepuce is still developing at this time and its separation is usually incomplete." Balanitis was another much-overworked diagnosis. In most cases labeled "balanitis," he maintained, the real problem was merely superficial inflammation of the foreskin, "usually due to ammonia dermatitis from ammoniacal urine." For such patients, he warned, "circumcision is strongly counterinidcated" because the foreskin protects the underlying glans.[20]

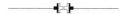

Opponents of circumcision have developed an anatomical portrait of the foreskin as a vital, dynamic, essential component of the male body. In their view, evolution is not inefficient; every facet of the normal body has its purpose. As a protective structure, the foreskin was best compared not with the fingernails, which need clipping to optimize the functioning of the fingers, but with the eyelid, a dynamic shielding layer that preserves the sensitivity of the eyeball. The sebaceous glands of the prepuce secrete smegma, a substance that lubricates the glans and keeps it moist. (Smegma was historically assumed to be a natural effusion of the body, analogous to the secretions produced by the vagina. As the prepuce became identified with disease, however, many within the Anglo-American medical community came to think of smegma as dangerous, or at least undesirable.)[21]

Protective functions aroused far less controversy than the erotic. Circumcision's real mischief, according to William Morgan, a Baltimore specialist in pulmonary medicine, was that it deprived men of sexual pleasure. For a man to experience sexual intercourse without a foreskin, he declared, was like viewing a Renoir color-blind.[22]

Since ancient times, as we have seen, most commentators—advocates and opponents alike—assumed that cutting off the foreskin dulled the libido. "There is not doubt that circumcision weakens the power of sexual excitement, and sometimes lessens sexual enjoyment," Maimonides wrote. "The organ necessarily becomes weak when . . . deprived of its covering." The foreskin itself is rich in nerves and nerve endings. Removing it certainly deprives a man of erogenous tissue and, some argue, "transforms the glans from an internal organ to an external one." Stripped of the prepuce, the glans, normally housed and lubricated by a layer of moist mucosal tissue, is exposed to the drier external environment and becomes comparatively scarified and insensitive. At the same time, the natural layer of keratin on the surface of the circumcised penis thickens. "The epithelium of the glans eventually becomes dry, dull, leathery, brownish, and keratinized," according to a physician opposed to circumcision, "taking on the character of skin rather than mucous membrane." Loss of sensitivity is in this view a continuing process, some older circumcised men complaining "that having intercourse with their circumcised glans is like having intercourse with their elbow."[23]

Critics also have noted that circumcision robs the penis of a dynamic element that contributes significantly to sexual pleasure. The mechanics of sexual activity—masturbation, foreplay, intercourse—involve ranges of motion: touching, gliding, expanding, contracting. The normal lubrication and sliding movement associated with the foreskin is simply missing if a man has been circumcised. Some physicians contend that women suffer as well. "Nature has designed it so that the female partner is stimulated by pressure and not friction," writes Paul M. Fleiss.

> The natural penis is self-lubricating. Vaginal secretions serve only to ease the initial insertion of the penis. Preputial secretions enable the foreskin to evert and revert smoothly over the glans. . . . Without the mobile sheath of the foreskin, the circumcised penis acts like a ramrod in the vagina. This is unnatural and has negative health consequences for women.

Hazards include abrasion, small ruptures and tears in the vaginal wall, in some instances producing bleeding and severe pain. To compensate for the lack of natural lubrication, many people resort to chemical substances whose long-term effects are unknown.[24]

To clarify what had been a narrow, monochromatic understanding of the foreskin, a team of Canadian pathologists led by J. P. Taylor from the University of Manitoba decided to subject samples of "the type and amount of tissue missing from the adult circumcised penis" to histological examination. As pathologists, these researchers had the opportunity to collect at autopsy the prepuces of twenty-two adult males between twenty-two and fifty-eight years old, and four circumcised babies (whose deaths were unrelated to circumcision).[25]

Like most anatomists dating back to Galen, the Canadian team viewed the prepuce as an integral part of the male genitalia. This conforms to common sense; in uncircumcised males the skin tissue covering the shaft of the penis is continuous, unbroken by any distinct border that defines the prepuce as a separate structure. Altogether, the penis impressed them with its complexity, and with the coordination of its specialized parts. Within this system, the prepuce is not just a fleshy cover. It serves as a platform for nerves and nerve endings. Indeed, the density of nerve fibers, particularly in the outer skin of the prepuce, make it as sensitive to light touch—and to pain—as any other part of the organ. The researchers found that the glans, usually assumed to be the most sensitive part, is comparatively less sensitive to light touch, heat, cold, and even to pinprick.[26]

The most remarkable feature of the prepuce had to do with the differences between its inner and outer surfaces. Its exterior is like the skin that covers much of our bodies. Its inner lining, however, is a type of skin found in only a few places in human anatomy: "variably-keratinized squamous epithelium similar to frictional mucosa of the mouth, vagina and esophagus." This smooth, moist epithelial tissue is a thicket of minute nerves, Schwann cells (associated with the myelin sheath around nerve fibers), lymphoid cells, and capillaries. Tiny protuberances called *papillae* stud the cell surface, and there are microscopic bundles of nerve endings that again resemble those in the inner lining of the mouth. Unlike the surface skin of the penis, which becomes toughened by exposure to the elements, the prepuce's inner mucosa never forms a dense collagenous layer. In addition, it remains entirely free of lanugo hair follicles, sweat, and sebaceous glands. The tissue is quickened by smooth

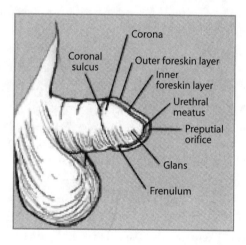

Neonatal penis.

muscle bundles of a type common to the skin on the penile shaft and preputial mucosa.

Examining the inner lining of the retracted foreskin from its tip down, the Canadian researchers described two regions: a narrow, ridged area some 10 to 15 millimeters wide merging into a larger, smooth one. Under high-powered magnification, the ridged mucosa reveal a pebbled or coral-like texture. In adult males, when the penis is relaxed and the prepuce unretracted, this ridged band is inverted, lying flat against the glans. During erection or when the prepuce is manually pulled back, the band is turned inside out on the shaft of the penis. The study's authors went on to assert that the ridged band—the skin that doctors would normally notice when examining the uncircumcised penis—misled the medical profession into thinking the entire foreskin was just ordinary skin. After all, "it is clearly visible on inspection of the retracted prepuce, it is continuous with the wrinkled true skin of the tip of the prepuce, and it looks like skin."

Yet in this instance, the researchers claimed, looks are deceptive. The ridged band is more like the skin of the lips, forming a transition between the facial skin and the mucosa inside the mouth. Regions of the body where such junctions occur, the argument goes, are worthy of special attention. Indeed, previous anatomists had described "mucocutaneous end-organs" or "genital corpuscles" in the glans penis and foreskin resembling the oval, encapsulated sensory nerve endings first described by the German physiologist Georg Meissner. These distinctive corpuscles of the prepuce should be compared to similar nerve endings in the fingertips and lips, they concluded, "which respond in a fraction of a second to contact with light objects that bring about deformation of their capsules."

The striking conclusion Taylor and his colleagues reached is twofold. The prepuce itself is a physiologically complicated structure with specialized parts that serve different functions. The "ridged band," for example, is made up primarily of sensory tissue whose neural structure differs from that of the glans. Presumably, in the dynamic flow of sexual activity, its contributions to sensation are unique. During erection, according to this dynamic model, the smooth mucosal inner lining and the outer true skin of the prepuce cooperate to "deploy" the ridged band, moving it down onto the shaft of the penis where its sensitive qualities come into play. They suggest that perhaps the conventional picture of the foreskin as a wrap protecting the glans should be reversed. "It is equally likely that the glans shapes and protects the prepuce," they speculate, with the ridged band working not only to intensify sensation but to help regulate the ejaculatory reflex.[27]

Yet the anatomy of Eros is hardly a precise science. Sexual sensation and pleasure involve much more than the physical stimulation of nerve endings. While it is possible to measure the tissue lost to circumcision, it is impossible to calculate the loss of pleasure, if any.

Their exploration of the prepuce convinced the Canadian pathologists to speak out publicly against circumcision, with Taylor becoming a popular presenter at anticircumcision forums. In addition, they proposed further research to investigate the function of the infantile prepuce. This had been peripheral to their study, but they observed that in early life the organ contains "muscle bundles, blood vessels and nerves in profusion; its internal organization is poorly understood but a case can be made for sensory tissue with the rigidity and form associated with specific function."[28]

So far, however, the "use" of the infant foreskin has meant mainly the use of the severed tissue after circumcision: ironically, in light of the mystical powers once attributed to the foreskin, modern molecular biology has discovered that it does indeed possess certain powerful, unexplained qualities. In the early 1990s, researchers at biotechnology companies happened on unexpected uses for the discarded prepuce. Scientists at Advanced Tissue Sciences (ATS) in California and at Organogenesis and BioSurface Technology in Massachusetts, engaged in the study of wound healing, developed techniques for culturing human epidermal tissue using neonatal foreskin cells called *fibroblasts*. From a single foreskin no larger than a postage stamp ATS could produce 250,000 square feet of Dermagraft, a bioengineered skin replacement product. "With one foreskin, you can grow about six football fields worth of skin through current cell culture techniques," explained Marie Burke of ATS. For reasons still poorly understood, foreskin cells are an ideal source of new biocompatible skin. So far it has been tested with some success on burn victims and patients suffering from diabetic foot ulcers. Unlike skin from another human, bioengineered tissue is not rejected by the body's immune system. Dermagraft has no blood vessels; the patient's own vessels migrate into the new tissue to nourish its growth. The cultured tissue forms the lower layer of skin, forming a base for the growth of epidermis. Meanwhile, a Texas company called Life-Cell Corporation managed to grow foreskin keratinocytes into a universal dermal tissue graft, a layer of "cultured dermis" that was successfully grafted onto experimental animals. "Wound healing is such a complex medical problem, no one knows what factors"—let alone in what amounts—can promote it, explained one BioSurface executive. "But the [fibroblast] cells are programmed to produce various factors so we don't have to answer those questions."[29]

SIX

Circumcision and Disease:

The Quest for Evidence

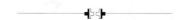

There are in fact two things, science and opinion; the former begets knowledge, the latter ignorance.

—*Hippocrates (460–377 B.C.)*

WHETHER OR NOT CIRCUMCISION MAKES MEN HEALTHIER IS A QUESTION THAT would seem to lend itself to a straightforward scientific answer. Yet if medicine is, in Lewis Thomas's apt phrase, "the youngest science," it is also the least precise.

The trouble is, theories based on careful accumulation of data may be confounded by an exceptional case. Inexplicably, some cancer patients experience spontaneous remission. Realizing this, doctors rely heavily on personal judgment. Medical knowledge of an individual patient is not superior to scientific knowledge; it is a different order of knowing, a kind of imaginative insight. In practice, by and large, physicians value experience over science.

The principles of cause and effect, of predictability, of precise experimental replication—in other words, much of what a chemist or physicist takes for granted—apply only loosely or metaphorically to medical science. In a typical drug study (called a *randomized controlled trial*), 200 people with, say, arthritis enroll to test a new pain medication. They are assigned to two groups: half are given the active compound, the other half a sugar pill placebo. No patient, nurse, or doctor involved in the study knows which is which. When the results

come in, it turns out that 43 percent of the group who received the real medicine experienced a measurable benefit; but so did 31 percent of those who
swallowed the placebo. The experiment is tried again, this time with 1,000
people, and the results are roughly the same. What conclusions should one draw
about the effectiveness of the drug? This kind of study, despite its vexing im-
precision, is the gold standard for evaluating new medicines. As we will see, it
is also a standard that no research into the health consequences of circumcision,
or most commonly performed surgeries, for that matter, has ever remotely approached.

Even calculating the basic rate of circumcision in the United States is hard
to do with accuracy. For some procedures, such as cardiovascular bypass grafts,
hospitals and physicians have maintained careful records; but the notion that
circumcision is trivial has discouraged systematic efforts to track it. For 1985,
the National Center for Health Statistics (sampling only a small percentage of
hospitals) estimated that 59.5 percent of American male infants were circumcised. There was significant variation by region: in the Northeast, 65.2 percent; in the Midwest, 70.6 percent; in the South, 56.1 percent; in the West,
49.0 percent. Meanwhile, researchers in New York, using similar sampling
techniques, estimated that 45.5 percent of boys born in New York City and
69.9 percent of those born elsewhere were circumcised.[1]

Statistics like these underestimate actual practice. From 1985 to 1986, a
team of Atlanta researchers inspected the records of fifteen area hospitals to
see whether sensational local media reports of a few bad complications had
influenced doctors or patients. In the period of their survey, the rates decreased
from 89.3 percent to 84.3 percent, though they had no way of knowing
whether or not this drop was a reaction to the bad publicity. They did discover factors that, if taken at face value, would cause circumcision rates to
be underestimated. For 15.7 percent of circumcised boys, the procedure was
unaccountably omitted from their medical records; and for Jewish boys who
went home before they were eight days old, the bris was not noted by the
hospital.[2]

During the 1990s, the National Center for Health Statistics improved its
sampling procedures and methods of data collection. Estimated rates through
1996 are shown in Table 6.1.

In 1996, there were just under 2 million male births in the United
States, and perhaps 1.2 million circumcisions. These included four out of
five white male infants, two out of three blacks, but just over half of Hispanic
boys.[3]

PERCENTAGE OF U. S. INFANTS CIRCUMCISED			
	1994	1995	1996
Northeast	69.6	68.3	66.7
Midwest	80.1	79.8	81.0
South	64.7	66.1	63.6
West	34.2	42.6	36.2
Nationwide	62.7	64.1	60.2

TABLE 6.1

In a sense, Americans have conducted a unique, uncontrolled surgical experiment that, were its results known, could tell us a great deal about the relationship between circumcision and health. And there would seem to be a mountain of evidence. Since 1870, when Lewis Sayre issued his influential paper, medical periodicals have printed more than four thousand papers pertaining to circumcision. Professional journals, though, are a slippery medium for evaluating the success or failure of medical practices; they tend to confirm, not challenge, standard practice.

In the American system of private insurance, payers automatically covered the costs of the procedure based on physician consensus that it was medically beneficial. Not until the 1960s, in a period of intense challenges to received wisdom and institutional authority, did American doctors seriously question the legitimacy of routine neonatal circumcision. Why was it, asked the editors of the *Journal of the American Medical Association* in 1963, that an operation so well accepted by practitioners for its power to " 'relieve' phimosis, to 'prevent' infection, to be 'prophylaxis' against carcinoma" had attracted no interest from the medical research establishment?

Over the next several years, practitioners increasingly engaged their colleagues in debates about the procedure. Their arguments represent a mixture of epidemiology, opinion, prejudice, and cultural speculation. For instance, castigating circumcision as "the rape of the phallus," a physician at the University of Maryland blamed its popularity on women. "Perhaps not least of the reasons why American mothers seem to endorse the operation with such enthusiasm," he wrote, "is the fact that it is one way an intensely matriarchal society can permanently influence the physical characteristics of its males."[4]

A more thoughtful critique appeared in 1969 in the *New England Journal of Medicine*. In an article titled "Ritualistic Surgery—Circumcision and Tonsillectomy," pediatrician Robert Bolande insisted that there was insufficient evidence to justify any surgery as a preventive measure, and that cutting in the absence of disease violated the tenet of "first, do no harm." Many physicians have compared circumcision with tonsillectomy as examples of surgical fads. The need for tonsillectomy often seemed to depend more on the attitude of the doctor than the condition of the patient. In a famous experiment conducted in 1934, for example, New York City public health officials decided to see what doctors would say about the need for tonsil surgery in a random sample of 1,000 eleven-year-olds enrolled in the city schools. Of this group, 611 already had tonsillectomies. When the other 389 children were sent to community physicians for evaluation, surgery was prescribed for 174 (44.7 percent) of them. The remaining 215 children were then sent to a different group of doctors for evaluation, resulting in 99 (46.0 percent) more recommendations to operate. This left 116 who were in turn sent to yet another panel of doctors, who urged tonsillectomy in 51 (44.0 percent) cases. If doctors were evenly divided about the need for a preventive procedure, second and third opinions merely reflected the prevailing attitudes of the medical community. The condition of the patients was largely irrelevant.[5]

The closer physicians looked at the medical literature on circumcision, the more many wondered whether its supposed medical benefits could withstand scrutiny. The best that could be said, declared a writer in the *Journal of the American Medical Association*, was that "circumcision is a beautification comparable to rhinoplasty." In 1971, unable to find compelling data to the contrary, the American Academy of Pediatrics officially concluded that there were no medical grounds for routine infant circumcision, a decision it recanted in 1985 then reconfirmed in 1999 after exhaustive analysis of the medical literature. Meanwhile, Benjamin Spock, the famous pediatrician whose best-selling medical guide for parents had originally endorsed circumcision, changed his mind. Considering the findings of modern science, he reported, the operation was "unnecessary and at least mildly dangerous."[6]

Neither Spock's nor the Academy's position made much difference in medical practice. One reason is that the American Academy of Pediatrics (AAP), worried about dissent within its own membership, did not promote its decision. Also, during the same period the American College of Obstetricians and Gynecologists, whose members advised mothers on childbirth and themselves performed hundreds of thousands of circumcisions annually, refused to go along with the pediatricians. After several years of internecine quarreling, the *American Journal of Obstetrics and Gynecology* at last issued an opinion, albeit *sotto voce*. Although some studies found that circumcision facilitates hygiene, prevents local inflammation of the glans, and may reduce risk of carcinoma of the penis, declared the journal, other factors weighed against the operation. These included illogical bases for patient selection, lack of informed consent, disregard for pain, the performance of a radical technique by doctors unskilled in surgery, unclear clinical objectives, and no evidence for cost-effectiveness. "Clinicians ought to use techniques only when certain that they do good," was the conclusion. "In clinical practice physicians should not have to prove that techniques are not dangerous."[7]

The argument over the benefits of circumcision—the power of the operation to prevent various disorders—is fascinating in part because it illustrates the relationship between what is known from clinical research and what physicians actually do in the clinic. The argument also exposes the substantial difficulty of evaluating preventive measures. Considering that the United States devotes nearly 15 percent of its national income to health care, outcomes research that endeavors to quantify the risks and benefits of what doctors do in the clinic is a surprisingly primitive field.[8] With most medical tests and treatments, from mammography to cardiac surgery, the challenges of collecting, evaluating, and interpreting medical evidence mean that studies are seldom conclusive. At best, medical researchers speak in terms of strong probabilities. Even the most compelling study typically ends with a call for more research to confirm its findings. According to Marcia Angell, editor of the *New England Journal of Medicine*, "We can rarely absolutely prove a hypothesis, although we can gather enough evidence from enough different studies to make the hypothesis so probable that we can say it is true for all practical purposes."[9]

Adding to the problem of appraising medical evidence, as we have already noticed, is the notorious placebo effect. A placebo (Latin for "I shall please") is a sham medicine or treatment, sometimes dispensed to placate a worried patient for whom there is no appropriate intervention. The baffling part is that in many cases, the placebo brings about a powerful healing effect. Although most people think of placebos in terms of pharmaceuticals—sugar pills that mimic drugs—the effect is just as pronounced in surgery. A group of orthopedic surgeons in Texas, for example, conducted a study of arthroscopic surgery in patients who complained of severe knee pain. They randomly divided subjects into three groups: one that received surgery to scrape the knee joint; one whose joints were washed (a less invasive procedure); and finally, one group in whom the joint was left alone. To ensure that patients couldn't tell what had been done, the no-surgery group was given anesthesia, and while unconscious, superficial incisions were made in patients' knees. Disconcertingly, two years after the initial experiment, all three groups reported the same level of improvement, with substantially less soreness and swelling. Researchers have observed similar results from placebos in everything from baldness remedies to lung function in asthmatic children. "We are misled by dualism or the idea that mind and body are separate," remarked neuroscientist Howard Fields. The consequences of a surgery are not a mechanistic product of cutting, but a complex interplay of the procedure and the patient's expectations of its effects.[10]

Moreover, the consequences of surgery are not a product of the patient's expectations alone. Dan Molerman, a medical anthropologist, put it this way: "The physician is an agent for optimism and hope and a great inducer of beliefs." No doctor is an island. Study after study has shown that physicians and patients sway each others' perceptions. When several years ago results came in from a large controlled trial demonstrating that a popular drug for angina was actually no more effective than placebo, the drug's effectiveness sharply declined. In ways that are only beginning to be described, placebo dynamics seem to be linked not simply to the physicians but also influenced by particular cultures. Doctor Molerman discovered this when he compared 122 double-blind placebo-controlled ulcer studies from around the world. Compared to pharmaceuticals, placebos ranged from zero to 100 percent effective, the key variable being the country. In Germany, placebos healed 60 percent of ulcers, more than double the rate in the United States, and ten times the rate in Brazil, where placebos worked just 6 percent of the time. "I don't have a hint of what is going on here," Molerman confessed. "I can only say that cultural differences affect ulcer treatments, even though ulcers are the same the world over."[11]

The problem is to determine whether there is enough information of adequate quality to allow us to draw confident, robust conclusions. Applying scientific methods to neonatal circumcision poses unusual problems. Unlike most surgeries (cosmetic procedures are the obvious exception), circumcision is performed in the absence of disease. Any health benefits are not apparent until years, perhaps decades, later. Advocates are fond of saying that the pain of circumcision is momentary but its benefits accrue over a lifetime. Still, the ultimate question of whether the procedure does more good than harm to the patient's body, or for that matter, whether it does any good at all, is not a matter of faith or surmise but of biological fact.

The evidence that does exist falls into two basic categories. The first pertains to the immediate risks and complications of the surgery itself. The second concerns the effect circumcision may have on a male's propensity to suffer a variety of disorders later on. In both of these areas, the peer-reviewed medical literature on circumcision is riddled with contradictions.

RISKS AND COMPLICATIONS

Circumcision is an invasion of the body that automatically carries certain risks. "The way things go wrong in medicine is normally unseen and, consequently, often misunderstood," according to physician and medical writer Atul Gawande. "Mistakes do happen. We think of them as aberrant; they are anything but." The behind-closed-doors nature of surgery (with the exception of bris ceremonies, few laypeople have ever witnessed a circumcision) means that the whole sense of risk is baffled and abstract. Even for specialists, weighing these risks is hardly an exact science. Procedures that do more harm than good are commonplace in the history of medicine. Ancient physicians bored holes through patients' skulls in the hope of releasing malignant spirits. As recently as 1949, the Portuguese neurologist Egas Moniz shared the Nobel Prize in medicine for pioneering the now-discredited frontal lobotomy.[12]

"Circumcision, one of the most common minor operations, is bunglingly done in many instances, notwithstanding its simplicity," observed Dr. S. L. Kistler in 1910. "Many a surgeon has lost his best clients, and likewise many a good prospect has gone glimmering because of the unfortunate outcome of this little operation." While the rate of major complications is certainly very low, there are scattered reports of medical misadventures: lacerations of the penile shaft, injuries to the glans caused by clumsy attempts to separate preputial adhesions, unintentional insertion of a scissors blade into the urethra, "bivalving the glans," and the loss of the penis from a doctor's foolishly using a rubberband as a tourniquet.[13] In a notably comprehensive survey, a review committee of the Canadian Paediatric Society remarked that "the prevalence of postoperative complications is unknown," though these complications included "easily controllable bleeding, amputation of the glans, acute renal failure, life-threatening sepsis and, rarely, death." Such complications would be apparent at the time of surgery, but as with many surgeries, circumcision may also produce adverse results that are not recognized until years later.[14]

The earliest methodical effort to reckon the medical risks associated with circumcision appeared in English pediatrician Douglas Gairdner's 1949 study, "The Fate of the Foreskin." Searching through the British Registrar-General's vital statistics for the years 1942 through 1947, he concluded that the procedure had claimed an average of sixteen children's lives annually. What went wrong? The main culprit in Gairdner's study—far more dangerous than the scalpel—was general anesthesia. "In most of the fatalities which have come to my notice," Gairdner wrote, "death has occurred for no apparent reason under anaesthesia, but haemorrhage and infection have sometimes proved fatal.... In my own experience about two out of every 100 children circumcised as hospital out-patients will be admitted on account of haemorrhages or other untoward event."[15]

General anesthesia was rarely used on infants in the United States. Compiling statistics based on hospital data in 1953, a pediatric researcher claimed that the complication rate in the United States was an infinitesimal 0.06 percent.[16] A much larger study, covering 100,157 boys circumcised in U.S. Army hospitals between 1980 and 1985, reported a somewhat higher (though still extremely low) incidence of complications: 0.19 percent. When doctors at the University of Washington Hospital sifted through the medical charts of 5,521 boys born in the 1960s and early 1970s, trying to compare outcomes associated with two competing circumcision devices, the Plastibell device and the Gomco clamp, they found that 59 patients (1.1 percent) had postoperative bleeding significant enough to merit special attention. In most cases, hemorrhage was traceable to anomalous blood vessels or to a bleeding disorder such as hemophilia. Indeed, circumcision in the hospital sometimes has been fatal to hemophiliac infants. Physicians have learned to intervene by supplying the missing coagulation factor in the form of local fibrin glue, rather than infusing a baby with clotting factor VIII concentrate.[17]

In several rare but widely publicized cases, attempts to control bleeding have resulted in disaster. In America and Britain, a common technique used to control surgical bleeding is known as electrosurgical diathermy, in which a forceps activated with electric current is used to cauterize tissue, sealing blood vessels. Unless the instrument is carefully controlled, however, the operator risks burning the patient. "At its most severe," according to a team of British physicians, "diathermy may result in total ablation of the penis." Researchers described four instances in which the damage was so extensive that repair was considered impossible. The results were chilling: "In all cases the children were managed by gender reassignment and feminizing genitoplasty."[18] In some cases, physicians ran into trouble because they experimented with medical devices neither designed for circumcision nor approved by the Food and Drug Administration for such use. In 1986, for example, a Louisiana jury awarded

$2.75 million to the family of a two-year-old boy whose penis was badly burned by a Louisiana State University medical resident. The damage was so severe that doctors asked the boy's parents to allow them to perform a sex change operation on him. The parents refused. Another such case occurred in 1985 in Atlanta's Northside Hospital that resulted in nationwide attention: a medical malpractice lawsuit yielded a spectacular damage award of $22.8 million. Because the hospital's normal equipment was out of service the day the boy was born, his physician used an electrosurgical device that was "contraindicated for use" in infant circumcisions. The plaintiff's attorneys argued that the boy would "never be able to function as a normal male and will require extensive reconstructive surgery and psychological counseling as well as lifelong urological care and treatment by infectious disease specialists."[19]

The chief criterion of a successful circumcision, whether medical or ritual, has always been aesthetic. The most common cause of cosmetic and functional problems is simply cutting too much or too little. If the surgeon fails to remove enough of the prepuce, the organ looks uncircumcised and the cultural significance of the operation is lost. Worse, in some cases the wound at the opening of the foreskin contracts, and as it heals forms a tough ring of scar tissue. Occasionally this fibrous ring shrinks back enough to cause phimosis; in extreme cases the constriction interferes with urination, requiring a second circumcision to restore normal function.[20]

Perhaps a more frequent error is for surgeons—especially inexperienced ones—to remove too much skin. This may happen if the foreskin is stretched too far over the glans when it is excised. After the operation, what is left of the prepuce slides back, leaving part of the penile shaft denuded. This problem usually resolves itself, though while new skin grows the patient is prone to infection. In litigious America, such mishaps invite lawsuits. In 1995, the Russian immigrant parents of a three-year-old boy won a $1.2 million settlement from a Brooklyn ambulatory surgical center. The parents sued the clinic, an attending physician, and the rabbi who performed the procedure for causing "permanent shortening and disfigurement of the penis." Expert witnesses at the trial testified that, owing to the disfiguring procedure, the boy was likely to encounter problems in sexual functioning when he reached maturity.[21]

Excising too much of the foreskin sometimes causes a condition known as *concealed penis*. This results when the surgeon removes too much of the outer prepuce but not enough of the foreskin's inner epithelial lining, which covers the glans penis. As the wound heals and contracts, the fibrous ring at the tip of the prepuce pushes the glans back into the suprapubic fat, leaving a small, ringed hole at the level of the skin in the mons pubis, with the penile shaft trapped subcutaneously behind it. A series of surgeries, including skin grafts, may be needed to correct this condition.[22]

To make the procedure foolproof, inventors have patented dozens of medical gadgets. Typical is the following weirdly incomprehensible abstract from a 1978 U.S. patent application.

> The device in its preferred form compresses in combination a male member which covers the head of the penis and has frictionally attached at one end a ring having an annular groove therein, a female member which fits over the shaft of the penis which compresses a plastic ring having a flexible wall such that its outside diameter can be increased or diminished in response to external compressive force exerted therein and therefrom.

At the beginning of the twenty-first century, the Plastibell device, the Gomco clamp, and the Mogen clamp remain the most popular instruments for circumcision. But as tools, they are only as good as those who use them. Even when they use these devices, physicians must accurately estimate the amount of skin to remove; they must forcibly separate the inner preputial epithelium from the epithelium of the glans; and finally, they must leave "the device in situ long enough to produce hemostasis," as the American Academy of Pediatrics Task Force on Circumcision put it, "and amputation of the foreskin."[23]

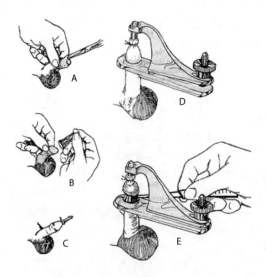

Circumcision using the Gomco clamp.

Pain

Mention of circumcision makes men wince. The penis is one of the body's most sensitive organs, and any sort of procedure on it is a harrowing prospect. Beyond the idea, however, how painful is circumcision truly? Do males cut in infancy experience the same kind of pain that older males feel? And if infants do feel acute pain, is it momentary and quickly forgotten, or does it have lasting effects? When is it appropriate to use anesthetics and analgesia, and which work best?

These are important questions. In deciding whether to undergo elective surgery, most adults weigh the expected pain against the benefit they expect. Babies are in no position to make a decision; but physicians, spurred by anti-circumcision activists, have in the past generation taken a fresh look at neonatal pain. Circumcision's popularity in America stems in large part from its transformation into a neonatal operation. For a man or a boy past infancy, surgery on the foreskin was frightening and recovery painful; newborns, in contrast, suffer no fear in advance of the operation. And doctors, who have long tended to underestimate (and undertreat) surgical pain, assumed that babies suffer little distress because their brains and nervous systems are undeveloped. Any distress they feel, the assumption ran, is fleeting. That *mohels* had circumcised eight-day-old infants for thousands of years with little evident trauma seemed to support these notions.

Measuring pain—especially in patients who cannot speak for themselves—is not easy. Before the 1980s, physicians and medical writers typically reassured anxious parents that cutting of the foreskin produced only momentary discomfort. As for their crying, according to a popular consumer medical guide published during the 1970s, infants naturally protested any prodding or restraint.

> Although the baby may scream and kick during the procedure, this seems to be more a reaction to being bundled to the circumcision board than actual pain. Many babies fall asleep during the process. Since a good portion of the baby's nervous system is not yet formed, especially that part that localizes pain, circumcision done at this age the first few days after birth is probably the best time.[24]

Some physicians, prominently anesthesiologists, dissented. "Circumcision without anesthesia is a cruel practice," declared the author of a popular consumer guide to child rearing in 1968. Pediatricians who studied infant pain produced unsettling descriptions of babies trembling, becoming "plethoric, dusky, and mildly cyanotic" because of their wailing, and on occasion, vomiting and breathing irregularly. Since circumcision usually is done within the first forty-eight hours after birth behind closed doors and out of sight of the infant's parents, the rate of minor complications is unknown. Still, there are occasional glimpses behind the veil. In one 1996 study of the effectiveness of local anesthesia, for instance, one baby in the group who was circumcised without anesthesia experienced a "serious postsurgery event."

> During and following circumcision, the newborn reacted much the same as others who received a placebo (continuously elevated heart rate and high-pitched cry). About 2.5 minutes after the conclusion of surgery, the newborn had an episode that included abnormal posture (lack of tone in limbs), several periods of apnea (one lasting more than 25 seconds), and projectile vomiting.

The researchers noted that another child in the placebo group had "a choking episode with apnea" after surgery.[25]

In 1987, researchers at the Harvard Medical School and Boston's Children's Hospital published a watershed paper in the *New England Journal of Medicine* in which they observed that pain pathways, along with the cortical and subcortical centers essential to pain sensation, are in fact well developed in the newborn child. They advised the medical community to take pain as seriously in infants as they would in older children and adults. Indeed, some commentators, such as Penelope Leach, wondered whether the experienced pain of circumcision was also remembered, leaving a permanent scar on the child's personality.[26]

At length, the American Academy of Pediatrics issued a policy statement on neonatal anesthesia. Specifically, they addressed the assumptions, held by many physicians, that anesthesia posed an unwarranted degree of risk to newborns, that babies' nervous systems were not developed enough to transmit pain, and that "neonates do not have sufficiently integrated cortical function to recall painful experience." Anesthesia had improved, the AAP said, so that local anesthetics could be applied without undue risk. They acknowledged that longstanding views of brain and neural pathway development in very young children were being revised in ways that suggested pain was as much a matter of concern for neonates as for adults.[27]

The AAP position resulted from convincing studies that closely monitored newborns before, during, and after surgery. As one might expect, the operation triggered significant physiological changes: in breathing, crying, heart rate, and cortisol levels. Immediately after the operation, babies demonstrated classic responses to intense stress: their appetites deteriorated and they became apathetic, disinclined to interact with their mothers or nurses. In some instances, circumcised infants needed to be fed infant formula, a finding that bothered some physicians, because early feeding with formula tends to reduce the duration of maternal breast-feeding.[28]

Not until 1994 did a well-designed study assess the pain of circumcision and the medical profession's inadequacy in dealing with it. A team of researchers at Rochester General Hospital in upstate New York, led by Cynthia R. Howard, conducted a prospective, randomized, double-blind, placebo-controlled clinical trial that involved measuring circumcision pain and finding out whether Tylenol (acetaminophen), a common treatment in hospitals, mitigated it. They used an especially interesting framework for gauging pain: it included changes in infants' heart rates, breathing, intensity and duration of crying, consolability, sociability (e.g., "eye contact, response to voice, smile, real interest in face"), motor activity, flexion of fingers and toes, and sleep patterns. Based on these indices, the team concluded that "circumcision causes severe and persistent pain," and that Tylenol had no effect on pain response during or immediately after the operation, though it did provide some benefit after six hours. The most likely explanation, they reasoned, was that circumcision pain was simply too severe to be relieved by a mild analgesic.[29]

Convincing as this research would seem, the medical profession's response has been sluggish. In 1978, physicians discovered they could apply the technique of penile dorsal nerve block in circumcision by injecting the anesthetic lidocaine immediately before cutting off the foreskin. While the claim of the pioneers of this technique to have rendered the procedure completely "painless" is questionable, there is no doubt that the anesthetic considerably dampened infants' pain and cortisone responses. Yet long after the introduction of this technique, most doctors continued to perform circumcisions without using any anesthesia at all. Why? Some claimed that superior skill, cutting quickly and cleanly, minimized the patient's discomfort. Others, including the circumcision advocate Edgar J. Schoen, worried that nerve block anesthesia caused local bruising and occasionally systemic reaction. He felt that a sugar-flavored pacifier and liquid Tylenol generally provided enough relief. A Minnesota study of the penile nerve block technique showed that many physicians simply did not understand pain in neonates or doubted the power of local anesthesia to eliminate it. Comparatively few had received training in how to apply the anesthetic. There was also reluctance to ask parents to give their consent for the application of anesthesia. In a Canadian survey of Ontario physicians, even though most respondents acknowledged that neonates feel and remember circumcision pain, they were unmotivated to learn about anesthetics, including the penile nerve block.[30]

More recently, there have been studies comparing the range of local anesthetics available: dorsal penile nerve block, "ring block," and a mixture of local anesthetics applied to the skin (EMLA). Using more precise methodology than previous researchers, one team found that the infants in their study who did not receive anesthetic "suffered from great distress during and following the circumcision, and they were exposed to unnecessary risk (from choking or apnea)." To critics who suggested that the pain of an injection in the penis was equal to the pain of the procedure itself, they produced data that showed otherwise. Of the three anesthetics studied, they declared ring block clearly superior. According to all test criteria, infants receiving ring block did not exhibit pain behavior even during the cutting and separation of the prepuce from the penis. In contrast, dorsal penile nerve block proved only partially effective. Least effective (though possibly better than nothing) was EMLA, perhaps because the anesthetic cream failed to penetrate deeply enough into sensitive tissue.[31]

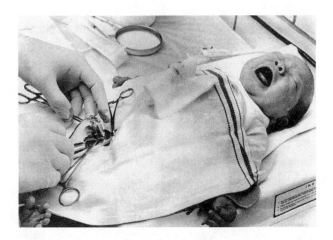

Routine neonatal circumcision.

Since most circumcisions are done without anesthetic, most boys suffer acute pain. Whether or not this pain makes a lasting impression—influencing the child's future development—has been hotly debated. A suggestive assessment of the later effects of circumcision pain was made by a group of Toronto physicians and psychologists who conducted a prospective study of children returning to the clinic for their four- and six-month vaccinations. Their notable finding was that circumcised infants demonstrated greater response to vaccination pain than did those whose foreskins were intact. This observation indicates that the early experience of pain may provoke biochemical changes in the way circumcised children's neural systems process painful stimuli. In effect, the original cutting sends signals to the spinal cord, inducing "a sustained state of central neural sensitization or hyperexcitability." They suggested that early traumas like circumcision might affect the mechanisms by which certain amino acids, neuropeptides, and receptors interact to transmit messages, perhaps permanently changing the body's response to pain. Furthermore, speculating far beyond what their data showed, the authors wrote that infants circumcised without anesthesia could suffer from post-traumatic stress syndrome "triggered by a traumatic and painful event and re-experienced under similar circumstances of pain during vaccination."[32]

CIRCUMCISION AND DISEASE

Medical research confirms our common sense that cutting an infant's penis is painful, though the implications of this pain for an individual's later development are hotly disputed. Nevertheless, the larger question about circumcision, as with any clinical intervention, is whether it improves patients' health. "There are indeed definite indications for circumcision," observed a team of academic medical center researchers, "but none is present in the newborn."[33] So the questions about circumcision are about the future: Does it yield longer life, less disease or disability? Does it improve function? Does it alleviate fear or anxiety? And if it does confer benefit, does the benefit outweigh the harm? In an era of managed care, there is also the inevitable question of whether the health benefits, if any, are worth the costs.[34]

In preventive medicine, the general rule is that the intervention should match the risk. When the risk is large, aggressive interventions make sense. The smaller the risk, the more caution one should exercise. Most preventive measures (with a few exceptions such as vaccinations and stopping smoking) produce minimal individual gains. The incidence of some diseases—cancer of the penis, for example—is tracked fairly closely. Others, such as phimosis or balanitis, are seldom tracked. One estimate holds that as many as 18 percent of uncircumcised boys may develop one of these latter conditions before they are eight years old.[35] Older youths may suffer "puberty induced phimosis," an inability to retract the foreskin smoothly and comfortably when the penis becomes erect. During puberty, the penis grows rapidly, and in boys with a long prepuce, the distal part of the prepuce sometimes fails to grow enough to allow the enlarged glans easily to pass back and forth. In many cases, the prepuce skin doesn't stretch out; it tears, creating scar tissue, which aggravates the problem.

The inner lining of the foreskin is an area where bacteria and fungal infections can grow. Inflammation of the glans is called *balanitis*. When the inner lining of the prepuce is inflamed, the term is *posthitis*, and *balanoposthitis* when the inflammation involves both glans and foreskin. For more than a century, British physicians thought of balanitis as a disease of hot, humid climates. Shipping company doctors often advised merchant seamen, particularly those who worked below decks in the engine room, to have themselves circumcised as a preventive measure. In some instances, chronic balanitis has been associated with excessive washing, particularly with strong soaps that may irritate sensitive tissue. Most often, though, it results from a microbial agent. Sometimes the inflammation becomes acute, with discharges of pus resembling gonorrheal infection. Repeated attacks can cause scarring of the glans and foreskin. Eventually, in extreme cases, the preputial tissue may toughen and compress, resulting in phimosis, as well as narrowing of the urethral opening (meatal stenosis). Thus phimosis and balanitis are related. Inflammation from balanitis makes the prepuce and glans tender; hygiene suffers, producing more irritation and inflammation that in turn causes scarring, thereby aggravating the phimosis. *Thrush balanitis* is an infection passed from women to men. Diabetics are prone to balanitis owing to increased levels of sugar in their urine. Penile warts, caused by virus, are more common in men with foreskins.[36]

CERVICAL CANCER IN WOMEN

Just as physicians attributed comparatively low rates of syphilis and gonorrhea in Jewish communities to circumcision, they made the same inference about the low incidence of cervical cancer among Jewish women. In the years after World War II, as concern about cancer grew in the industrialized democracies, fear spread that women whose sex partners were uncircumcised faced elevated risk. Writing in the *British Medical Journal* in 1947, for example, W. S. Handley guessed that the main cause of the disease was carcinogenic material transmitted to a woman from an uncircumcised man during sexual intercourse. Subsequent research, particularly a 1954 study published in the *American Journal of Obstetrics and Gynecology* and reported widely in the national press, lent weight to this notion. Subsequently, however, the study's author discovered that his research was invalid because many women in his sample did not know whether or not their husbands were circumcised. By the time he acknowledged his error, it was too late. His theory had become entrenched in the public domain. For many people both inside and outside the medical profession, it confirmed their prejudices and became an article of faith. When an enterprising physician named S. I. McMillen claimed in his best-selling book *None of These Diseases* that of 13,000 annual deaths from cancer of the cervix most could have been prevented "by following the instruction that God gave to Abraham," few thought to contradict him.[37]

Like all cancers, carcinoma of the cervix is a complex disease, the causes of which are far from clear. It generally strikes women between the ages of thirty-five and fifty-five. For unknown reasons, the risk appears to be greater as a woman's age of first sexual intercourse decreases and as her lifetime number of sexual partners increases. As oncologists have studied the disease, the question about circumcision has centered on the human papillomavirus (HPV) and whether this virus, sometimes transmitted during coitus, may cause some forms of cervical cancer.[38]

Cervical and penile cancers are in fact closely linked to HPVS. Yet the mechanism of cancer development also involves such biological factors as the vulnerability of different types of epithelial tissue to infection and the local response of an individual's immune system to HPVS. Some urologists have hypothesized that secretions beneath the foreskin may contain mutagens, substances that stimulate natural cellular mutation and thus may turn cervical cells precancerous. Still, whether these are factors in cervical cancer remains doubtful.[39]

According to the cesspool theory (epitomized in one pediatrician's assertion that "for millennia the male's preputial cavity has acted as a cesspool for infectious agents"), the inner surface of the foreskin is a breeding ground for HPVS. So it would stand to reason that removing it reduces the viral population and the associated risk. Against this idea, as Ronald L. Poland pointed out, "studies have correlated exposure to uncircumcised sexual partners with the incidence of cervical cancer, but the circumcised state is also associated with the presence of the human papillomavirus and other possibly oncogenic viruses." Epidemiology (the study of diseases within population groups) raises the greatest questions. While Jews still tend to have comparatively low cervical cancer rates, other circumcised populations (specifically Muslims and American Gentiles) do not. If circumcision were a significant variable, one would expect lower cervical cancer rates across America than, say, in Germany; but the rates are similar. More than a generation ago, two skeptical physicians evaluating women in a cancer detection clinic found that

> The discovery rate for cancer of the cervix among non-Jewish women whose marital partners were circumcised was no different from the rate among non-Jewish women with noncircumcised husbands. Further, the use of a sheath contraceptive by the marital partner, which has an effect equivalent to circumcision in that the cervix is protected from contact with the smegma, was not found to be associated with rate difference for cancer of the cervix.

Reviewing the literature going back more than forty years, in 1996 the Canadian Paediatric Society's Fetus and Newborn Committee concluded that "no specific cause-and-effect relation between exposure to uncircumcised sexual partners and cervical cancer has been established."[40]

CANCER OF THE PENIS

A malignancy that attacks the reproductive organs holds special terror for women and men alike. This explains why cancer of the penis, a very rare disease, figures so prominently in the circumcision debate. It first appears as a scaly patch of skin that doesn't heal. Sometimes it develops into a wartlike tumor that eventually changes into an open sore. Like many forms of cancer, cancer of the penis is not only dangerous as a local condition but also potentially fatal if it metastasizes.

The observation that penile carcinoma is almost unknown in circumcised men dates back to the late nineteenth century. In the modern era, an article by Abraham Wolbarst that appeared in the *Lancet* in 1932 reported that Jewish men, circumcised shortly after birth, were never hospitalized for cancer of the penis. Though little more than an unscientific rehash of earlier impressions and stereotypes, Wolbarst's paper lent an aura of legitimacy to the idea that circumcision prevented penile cancer. Yet to a urologist writing in 1935 it seemed obvious that a man's being uncircumcised might be a less significant risk factor than his health habits and hygiene. "Men with penis cancers gave the impression of being less intelligent, as a class, than other cancer patients.

Not only had the majority ignored for long periods the precancerous state of physical annoyance, filth, and odoriferous discharges, but also it was not unusual for many to delay seeking advice until a large part of the penis had become affected with an ulcerating growth."[41]

Still, for most of the twentieth century it was taken for granted that circumcision prevented penile cancer. The 1986 edition of *Campbell's Urology*, a standard medical text, declared that "any argument against circumcision must take into account that penile carcinoma represents the only neoplasm for which there exists a predictable and simple means of prophylaxis that spares the organ at risk." Describing the history of relevant research up to 1991, Edgar Schoen cited Dean's 1935 finding that of 120 cases of penile cancer at Memorial Hospital in New York City, none was circumcised.

> In the subsequent 56 years, published studies from U.S. medical centers have confirmed Dean's findings. There were reports of 139 penile cancers from Illinois in 1946; 100 from Roswell Park, New York, in 1972; 156 cases from Michigan in 1973; and 77 from Cleveland in 1986. Of the resulting 592 penile cancer cases from five institutions around the U.S., not one of the men had been circumcised in infancy despite the fact that by the mid-1970s most males in the U.S. had been circumcised as newborns.[42]

Even so, the evidence is contradictory. Over the past decade, data concerning penile neoplasms in circumcised men have surfaced to challenge this view.[43]

Fortunately, the disease is so uncommon that it is hard to study. In developed countries, incidence runs between 0.3 and 1.1 per 100,000 men per year. This compares to 3 to 7 cases annually per 100,000 men in developing nations. The overall rate in the United States is just under 1 per 100,000: that is, 9 or 10 cases annually per million men, only 0.16 percent of total cancers in American males. Most of these cases occur in uncircumcised men, among whom the rate is projected to be 2.2 per 100,000. While this is miniscule compared to heart disease or stroke, Thomas E. Wiswell (an advocate for circumcision) contends that the annual rate understates the total risk for an individual over his lifetime. According to this argument, if men live on average 75 years, the chances of a man contracting the disease are 75 in 100,000. (Employing Wiswell's logic, however, the actual chances would be lower, because penile carcinoma is virtually unknown in boys and young men.) Moreover, since the malignancies almost never strike circumcised men, the minority of

uncircumcised men—30 percent of the population, in Wiswell's estimate—
absorb virtually all of the risk. In his reckoning, this means that for uncircumcised American men the lifetime rate of penile cancer is 250 in 100,000, or
0.25 percent.[44]

The main objection to the theory that circumcision lowers the rate of penile cancer is that some countries where males are rarely circumcised have
lower cancer rates than the United States. Finland, for example, with a circumcision rate below 1 percent, reported in 1970 a penile carcinoma rate of
0.5 per 100,000. In Denmark, where the circumcision rate is about 1.6 percent, penile cancer has been in steady decline since World War II and now
runs well below that of the United States. Danish researchers found that men
who had never married had a higher incidence of penile cancer than their
control group, and speculated that, as for so many other diseases, low socio-
economic status was a risk factor. The simplest explanation for changes in the
modern rate may be that during the postwar period personal hygiene improved because the percentage of dwellings with a bath rose from 35 percent
in 1940 to 90 percent in 1990. Hygiene correlates with cancer risk.[45]

So, generally speaking, what is one to make of this risk?

At one extreme, a procircumcision medical writer suggested that parents
who decided *not* to circumcise should be required to sign a medical disclo-
sure form warning that unless the child takes meticulous care of his penis,
he faces increased chances of developing cancer. Alternatively, one urologist
calculated that because penile cancer is so infrequent, a doctor would have
to perform 140 circumcisions a week for twenty-five years to prevent just
one case.[46]

In 1993, researchers at Seattle's Fred Hutchinson Cancer Research Center
repeated the assertion that "epidemiological evidence suggests lack of neonatal circumcision as the strongest risk factor for penile cancer." In their sample
population, the risk for penile cancer was 3.2 times greater for uncircumcised
men than for those circumcised as infants. Curiously, for reasons nobody understood, men circumcised *after* the neonatal period had about the same risk
as those who were uncircumcised. Studies of groups in China and Africa indicate that circumcision after the neonatal period may even increase the statistical likelihood of penile cancer. Again, there is no good explanation for
why this should be so.[47]

Beyond circumcision, other factors—cigarette smoking, frequency and
type of sexual activity and number of partners, sexually transmitted diseases,
and medical conditions of the penis—seem to make the greatest difference.
For instance, smokers were at 2.8 times greater risk than for men who never

smoked tobacco. And men with histories of penile rashes or penile tears were at much higher risk. By implication, as the researchers knew, the larger question had to do with the complex "interrelationships of circumcision, infection with HPV, and smoking as risk factors."[48]

Indications that genital warts and HPV are associated with penile cancer may mean that elevated risk for the disease emerges from a set of factors, some physiological, some behavioral. It is plausible that HPV may correlate with the number of sexual partners a man has as well as his sexual practices. Smoking may be less a contributing factor in its own right than a marker of lower health awareness and a general ignorance of health risks. The question is: If uncircumcised men practiced different sexual health habits, would the rate change?

In any case, though, the evidence is conclusive that circumcision prevents penile cancer just as mastectomy prevents breast cancer. Removing one third to one half of the skin of the penis lowers the odds of contracting what is, after all, a skin cancer. A high percentage of skin cancers eventually develop on the nose, one dermatologist noted; but this has not led physicians to recommend prophylactic rhinoplasties.

When physicians at the American Cancer Society reviewed the data in 1996, however, they publicly discouraged "the American Academy of Pediatrics from promoting routine circumcision as preventative measure for penile or cervical cancer." Officially speaking, "The American Cancer Society does not consider routine circumcision to be a valid or effective measure to prevent such cancers." The Society's medical committee figured that fatalities from penile cancer we probably offset by fatalities from circumcision. More important, they felt that highlighting circumcision as a preventive measure might distract men from avoiding high-risk behavior such as cigarette smoking and unprotected sexual relations with multiple partners. In 1984 a group of Canadian physicians analyzed the tradeoffs between circumcision and cancer and concluded that, based on an incidence rate of two cases per 100,000 men annually, it would cost $3.8 million to prevent those two cases, roughly 100 times the cost of treatment.[49]

This cost-benefit analysis puts the debate in stark relief. For proponents of neonatal circumcision, performing 100,000 operations to prevent two cases of cancer seems entirely reasonable. Opponents consider this tradeoff wildly out of balance. In the United States, with its deep aversion to rationing medical care or making explicit judgments based on resources, no consensus exists about where to draw the line.

SEXUALLY TRANSMITTED DISEASES

During the European syphilis epidemic of the sixteenth century, the Italian anatomist Gabriello Fallopio remarked on a relationship between the foreskin and the disease. "Men with long foreskins and a covered glans can be contaminated [by syphilis] more easily because they are more tender," he observed, "and there receive the virus [*sic*] more readily." Among circumcised men, in contrast, "less than two in a thousand are infected with the French sickness."[50]

From Fallopio's time to ours, many physicians have believed that the foreskin increases a male's susceptibility to sexually transmitted diseases (STDs). In the wake of World War II, for example, *Newsweek* quoted Eugene Hand's address to the American Medical Association in which he declared that "promiscuous" and uncircumcised Negroes had an incidence of venereal infection of "almost 100% [whereas] the widely educated Jew," because he was "circumcised at birth" experienced a low and decreasing incidence of the same diseases. Hand based this remark on research that shows how little medical understanding had advanced since Fallopio's day.

> Venereal infection is less likely in the circumcised because of the physical and histologic changes that occur on the distal end of the penis after circumcision. . . . The skin of the corona, glans, frenulum and distal portion of the shaft in the circumcised is tough, keratinized, dry and a degree or more cooler than is the area under the prepuce of the uncircumcised. . . . Jews have universally been circumcised on the eighth day after birth. This procedure has given them protection against venereal disease even when they have been exposed. . . . Circumcision is not common among Negroes. . . . Many Negroes are promiscuous. In Negroes there is little circumcision, little knowledge or fear of venereal disease and promiscuity in almost a hornet's nest of infection. Thus the venereal rate in Negroes has remained high. Between these two extremes there is the gentile, with a venereal disease rate higher than that of Jews but much lower than that of Negroes.

In 1947, R. A. Wilson published figures demonstrating that among soldiers treated in a Canadian Army venereal disease clinic a disproportionate majority were uncircumcised: 77 percent versus 52 percent in the Canadian Army generally. Even at the time, though, a critic noted that "since circumcision of infants is *de rigeur* in Canada, the uncircumcised man will tend to come from a lower social grade and thus be more likely to expose himself to infection."[51]

The belief that circumcision protects against sexually transmitted diseases may be wishful thinking related to America's extraordinary national rate of diseases passed through sexual contact and the powerlessness of public health to do much about it. The United States leads the developed world in STDs. According to a recent Institute of Medicine study, more than one in five Americans may be infected with chlamydia, HIV, syphilis, gonorrhea, herpes, and hepatitis B. Comparisons to other countries are striking: in Sweden, for example, the rate of gonorrhea is 3 in 100,000; in Canada, 18 in 100,000; in the United States, 150 in 100,000. While the explanation for these enormous differences is complicated, it is clear that widespread opposition to sex education in schools and to practical preventive measures, such as distributing condoms, are important factors. Americans ignore the epidemic and gloss over the human behavior that fuels it.

Medical research on the relationship between circumcision and STD has been anything but conclusive. An Australian study in 1983, typical of many others, found significant associations—fourfold to fivefold—between being uncircumcised and being diagnosed with genital herpes, candidiasis, gonorrhea, and syphilis. Yet nothing was built into the study design to account for other factors that might influence whether or not a man contracted a sexually transmitted disease.[52]

A carefully controlled large-scale study of 2,227 professedly heterosexual men who visited a Seattle STD clinic in 1988 discovered mixed results. Uncircumcised men experienced a higher incidence of syphilis and gonorrhea, but they were less likely to have genital warts. As for genital herpes, chlamydia and nongonococcal urethritis, circumcision appeared to make no difference.* For syphilis, the researchers calculated that the odds of an uncircumcised man being infected were 4.0 times greater than for his circumcised counterpart. For gonorrhea, the odds dropped to 1.6 times greater, certainly still significant.[53]

The Seattle researchers couldn't say why the uncircumcised men in their study should have proved more susceptible to gonorrhea and syphilis. But they did offer several hypotheses: the foreskin may suffer microscopic tears during

---

*Nongonococcal urethritis—so called to distinguish it from infections caused by *Neisseria gonorrhoae*—is usually the work of tiny bacteria: *Chlamydia trachomatis* or *Ureaplasma urealyticum*. These are highly contagious, infecting men and women. In men, symptoms include a burning sensation during urination and discharges of fluid or pus. In two out of three cases, the symptoms spontaneously disappear within four weeks. In some untreated men, however, chlamydia produces epidiymitis, with painful inflammation of the scrotum.

sexual intercourse that open pathways for bacterial infection; the moist, protected area underneath the prepuce could harbor bacteria that would otherwise die, prolonging exposure to infection; the glans and preputial sac of an
uncircumcised male, being comparatively thin and tender, might pose a less
substantial barrier to bacilli; and balanoposthitis (inflammation of the penis or
foreskin typically originating from bacterial or yeast infection) may be more
common in uncircumcised men and may predispose them to additional microbial invasion.

The idea that the warm, moist environment beneath the foreskin fosters
infection has been repeated so often that many physicians take it for fact, but
there is scant evidence that this is so. Indeed, some research suggests the opposite. Mucosal tissue—the kind of skin found lining the prepuce and a few
other places in the body, such as the inside of the mouth—has special immune
properties that may actually decrease the risk of infection. According to one
researcher, "The prostatic, urethral, and seminal vesicle secretions, which are
rich in lytic material, lubricate the mucosal surface of the inner surface and
glans. There, secretions in combination with mucosal flora and secretory im-
munoglobulins may protect the uncircumcised man."[54]

That other STDs—including genital herpes and penile warts—didn't appear
to be associated with an intact foreskin (indeed, uncircumcised men appeared
to be 30 percent less likely to suffer from warts) left the research team questioning its own methods. A diagnosis of genital herpes, for instance, depended on
the presence of observable lesions. If foreskins concealed some lesions, they reasoned, the true rate of herpes infection among uncircumcised men could have
been underestimated. The finding concerning genital warts confused them, and
so they left it to a future paper to develop a suitable theory.[55]

The fact that the Seattle study only included men who chose testing or
treatment at a public health clinic—a high-risk population—limited the application of its conclusions. Plainly, this group did not represent the social,
economic, and cultural norms of the American male population.

To explore the effects of circumcision in the mainstream, a team of researchers led by Edward O. Laumann, a University of Chicago sociologist, endeavored to extract data from the 1992 National Health and Social Life
Survey (NHSLS). This survey is a rich source of information about the health,
attitudes, and sexual activities of Americans. Its strengths include a large randomized sample intended to be representative of the 150 million men and
women between the ages of eighteen and fifty-nine. In the survey, men were
asked whether they were circumcised (though not, alas, when the procedure

had been done). They also were asked whether a physician had ever told them that they were infected with an STD. Interviewers went through a list of diseases. Depending on the response of the subject, to make sure the questions were understood they also used slang names for certain diseases (e.g., *clap* for gonorrhea).[56]

What makes Laumann's investigation unusually interesting is that it not only considered the differences in STDs among circumcised and uncircumcised men but also brought in several other social and cultural factors, such as whether a man lived in a city or the country; his age, race, religion, and ethnic background; his self-assessed attitudes toward sex (rated on a seven-point scale from very liberal to extremely conservative); and most critically, the number of sexual partners during the course of his life. All these factors were included in a complex statistical analysis.[57]

When the analysis was applied to STDs, the investigators found that "circumcision serves as an independent variable rather than a dependent variable." This means that a man's circumcision status was not useful in predicting the likelihood of his having suffered an STD. According to their data, "circumcised men were slightly more likely to have had both a bacterial and a viral STD in their lifetime." And where older studies had failed to consider nongonococcal urethritis or chlamydia, Laumann found that more than 2 percent of circumcised men reported at least one bout of chlamydia, yet no uncircumcised men did. For men with a history of more than twenty sexual partners, circumcision correlated with a nearly threefold (2.88) increase in STDs. Thus broadly speaking, the team noted "with respect to STDs, we found no evidence of a prophylactic role for circumcision and a slight tendency in the opposite direction."[58]

CIRCUMCISION AND HIV

In the summer of 1996, Stephen Moses, a Canadian AIDS researcher affiliated with Kenya's University of Nairobi, shocked a conference of scientists by telling them that there was now a "substantial body of evidence" that male circumcision provided protection against HIV infection. Abstracting results from scores of studies, Moses calculated that uncircumcised men were between 1.5 and 9.6 times more likely to become infected with the virus than their circumcised counterparts. Perhaps, he conjectured, with a nod toward a map showing the global variability of the epidemic, circumcision "may explain part of the wide geographic and population-level variability in observed HIV transmission."[59] About the same time, *Scientific American* published an article entitled "The African AIDS Epidemic" in which the authors overlaid maps of sub-Saharan Africa showing the spread of AIDS, with maps showing the geography of circumcision. There appeared to be strong correlation: the areas with the lowest rates of circumcision showed the highest rates of AIDS. Could lack of circumcision, they asked, make men in certain regions especially vulnerable?[60]

AIDS is the most intensely studied infectious disease in history, and perhaps the most perplexing. Certainly if there is evidence that circumcision offers significant protection, the finding could have public health consequences, particularly in Africa and other developing regions where the contagion is widespread and medicine scarce.

HIV passes from one person to another through contact with body fluids—blood, semen, vaginal secretions, and so forth—that contain infected cells or particles of the virus. Researchers who maintain that circumcision has some preventive effect on HIV transmission have suggested four different theories: (a) since there is a strong correlation between STD infection and susceptibility to HIV, if one assumes that circumcision reduces the risk of STDs, it is logical to infer that circumcision reduces the risk of HIV; (b) the intact foreskin multiplies the area of tissue vulnerable to inflammation and minor rupture during intercourse, offering HIV a greater variety of pathways into the bloodstream; (c) in circumcised men, the outer layer of skin covering the glans penis grows tougher, with a protective layer of keratin serving as a sort of "natural condom"; (d) the ecology of the inner foreskin may foster the survival of HIV for longer periods, increasing the opportunities to transmit the infection.[61]

The foreskin has a rich and dynamic physiology that in the opinion of some investigators makes it a magnet for infection. "Because the foreskin is associated with high concentrations of macrophages and lymphocytes," one group reported in 1993, "these cells are targets for HIV virus." Others reached similar conclusions. "Male circumcision consistently shows a protective effect against HIV infection," a team of epidemiologists and infectious disease specialists wrote in the *New England Journal of Medicine* in 1997. "This may be due to the abundance of Langerhans' cells [skin cells that actively emigrate to local lymph nodes] in the foreskin or a receptive environment for HIV in the sulcus between the foreskin and glans."[62]

These theories are not wildly improbable, but weaknesses in the studies on which they are based make them impossible to validate. Some of these deficiencies are plain to see. The widely cited *Scientific American* article, for example, submits that the negative correlation between circumcision and AIDS in sub-Saharan Africa indicates a cause-and-effect relationship. Yet the same mapping technique applied to North America would reveal the opposite cor-relation. The United States has far higher per-capita rates of both circumcision and HIV infection than Canada, but no one has pointed to circumcision to explain the difference. Nor do the regional differences in American circumci-sion rates match up with the regional incidence of HIV.

An example of the kind of study that makes up much of the epidemio-logical literature on circumcision and AIDS is a paper published in 1996 in the *Journal of Acquired Immune Deficiency Syndrome and Human Retrovirology* enti-tled "High Rates of Sexual Contact with Female Sex Workers, Sexually Trans-mitted Diseases, and Condom Neglect Among HIV-Infected and Uninfected Men with Tuberculosis in Abidjan, Côte d'Ivoire." Essentially, the investiga-tors conducted a case-control study at two large tuberculosis treatment cen-ters over a period of three years, employing as their subjects 490 men who tested positive for HIV and 239 who were uninfected. In regard to circum-cision, the key finding was that men with foreskins were 2.22 times more likely to be infected with HIV than those without. Taken by itself, this seems to show that the foreskin is a serious risk factor. The trouble comes when one tries to isolate circumcision from other factors that bear on HIV infec-tion. In this case, confounding variables included sexual activity with prosti-tutes, genital ulcers, urethritis, and condom use. Circumcision is not random. It remains an expression of powerful cultural and religious ideas. Knowing this, we are apt to wonder whether the circumcised practice different hygiene, engage in different sexual behaviors, or even eat different foods than the uncir-cumcised.[63]

What confuses the issue even more is that although a majority of the ob-servational studies performed thus far support claims of modest risk reduction for HIV infection for circumcised men, some of the most carefully controlled do not. A large 1995 study in rural Tanzania enrolling 12,534 adults found that for HIV, "prevalence was higher in circumcised men, but not significantly after adjusting for confounders." Moreover, most studies to date have dealt with only one aspect of the problem: susceptibility. But even if circumcision does make a man less susceptible to contracting HIV, does it do anything to reduce the contiguousness of those already infected? Could circumcision ac-tually make them *more* infectious to female partners? Researchers have only begun to address these questions.[64]

If it turns out that circumcision does afford a minor degree of reduced risk, what are the practical consequences? One worry, of course, is that given the public's poor understanding of epidemiological risk in the first place, cir-cumcised men would take the news as permission to engage in high-risk behavior. Prevalent circumcision has not kept the United States from becoming the industrialized nation most afflicted by HIV. As for poorer nations, the prospect of implementing neonatal circumcision on a population basis is near zero. Genital cutting is an expression of culture. The hurdles the United Nations Food and Agriculture Organization has encountered around the world in trying to combat malnutrition by encouraging seemingly simple changes in farming techniques gives us a hint of how difficult it would be to teach people to operate on babies' penises as a preventive measure. As a matter of fact, the reasonable and well-intentioned efforts of the international public health community to eradicate female circumcision illustrates just how great the obstacles are.

Since the United States has already reaped whatever protection against HIV that circumcision may afford, it remains for Europe to ponder the impact on public health. With rapidly aging populations demanding increasing amounts of health care, Europeans are unlikely to welcome any measure sure to produce low benefits at high cost.

URINARY TRACT INFECTION

In the United States during the late 1970s and early 1980s, the intellectual winds appeared to have shifted against circumcision of newborns. The baby-boom generation was coming of age and having babies. Mothers and fathers who had grown up in the 1960s tended not to share their parents' deference to medical sovereignty. Likewise, younger doctors, abreast of the latest research, realized that the science supporting circumcision was equivocal at best. But just at the time it seemed fated to join tonsillectomy on the ash heap of popular operations no longer considered appropriate, a new rationale emerged: prevention of urinary tract infection (UTI). On this subject, a continuous stream of empirical evidence in support of circumcision flowed through the medical journals, where it encountered striking professional interest and acceptance. In 1993, Edgar Schoen, chairman of the Task Force on Circumcision of the American Academy of Pediatrics, called the accumulated evidence that circumcision reduces the rate of UTIs "conclusive." Considering its preventive power, he said, the operation ought to be determined "*analogous to immunization* in that side effects and complications are immediate and usually minor, but benefits accrue for a lifetime" (emphasis in original).[65]

The apostle of this argument was U.S. Army pediatrician Thomas Wiswell, stationed at the Brook Army Medical Center on Fort Sam Houston in Texas.

As a young doctor, according to his own account, he sided with the 1975 American Academy of Pediatrics Task Force on Circumcision, which declared that no medical indication existed for routine operations. And as one would expect, an inspection of military hospital records for the years following the task force report showed that circumcisions were being performed at a declining rate. What had gone unnoticed, until Wiswell and his colleagues brought it to national attention, was that as the circumcision rate dropped, the number of UTI cases in boys skyrocketed.[66]

Wiswell was familiar with a 1982 retrospective study of neonatal pyelonephritis in male infants that reported that 95 percent of patients with this diagnosis were uncircumcised. The authors had speculated that being uncircumcised increased a boy's susceptibility to urinary tract infections. Based on the data he gathered, Wiswell concluded that the incidence of UTIs was ten times greater in uncircumcised than in circumcised males. This was not an insignificant finding. Bacteria that cause UTIs in some cases could cause kidney disease or death from acute pyelonephritis and sepsis. In its acute form, pyelonephritis can lead to permanent renal scars that in an estimated 2 percent or 3 percent of cases eventually result in kidney failure. End-stage renal disease is rare in children and young people, but in 20 percent of those who do contract the disease, it emanates from recurrent bacterial infections. Wiswell suggested that in the 1970s UTIs were uncommon, but that the rate climbed in the 1980s, when comparatively fewer circumcisions were being performed. In his largest study, Wiswell and his colleagues considered a sample of 209,339 children born between 1985 and 1990 in U.S. Army hospitals around the world. Of these, 550 girls and 496 boys (a total in all of 1,046 or 0.5 percent) were hospitalized with UTIs during the first year of life. Within the group, uncircumcised boys had a tenfold greater incidence of UTI than did circumcised boys. Wiswell confirmed this finding by conducting a meta-analysis of nine previously published studies of the relationship between circumcision and UTI. "These studies revealed a five-fold to 89-fold increased risk of infection in uncircumcised boys; the combined data yielded a 12-fold increase in UTIs in this population."[67]

Questions have been raised about the validity of this data. How accurate was the reporting of circumcision status? The information was abstracted from military hospital records where, among other things, there was no need to flag circumcision in the patient's medical chart in order to trigger an insurance payment, because the procedure was done by salaried military doctors. Circumcision was so commonplace, according to some critics, that it was probably significantly underreported. Underreporting would overstate the incidence of UTIs among the uncircumcised population. And do children admitted to a hospital for UTI represent the larger population? What would the results look like if those treated in a doctor's office or went untreated were counted? Despite reasonable questions about Wiswell's methods, though, subsequent research has confirmed his basic finding. An Australian team at Sydney's Royal Alexandra Hospital for Children conducted a case-control, age-adjusted study between 1993 and 1995 involving 144 boys under the age of five years with diagnosed UTI compared to 742 boys who did not have UTI. Of the 144 boys with UTI only 2 were circumcised, compared to 47 of the 742 control subjects. They reasoned that uncircumcised boys were four to five times more likely to contract UTI than those who were circumcised. In 1999, the American Academy of Pediatrics Task Force on Circumcision, based on a comprehensive review of published medical literature, estimated that "7 to 14 of 1,000 uncircumcised male infants will develop a UTI during the first year of life, compared with 1 to 2 of 1,000 circumcised males."[68]

Wiswell has been successful in part because he presented himself as a skeptic, a scientist reluctantly coming to see the importance of circumcision only because the data were so compelling. Once converted, however, like Lewis Sayre a century earlier, he took up the scalpel and the pen with equal passion. Before long he became the bête noire of anticircumcision groups. "Several years ago when I worked in Washington, D.C.," he told an interviewer in 1997, "one of the groups had a police detective come to the hospital after me because they claimed I was mutilating genitalia." When the police realized they were interrupting a circumcision, they left. But Wiswell's paranoia remained. He learned to make hotel reservations under aliases, to schedule his medical society presentations on the last day of conferences, and routinely to request extra security.[69]

It is no mystery why Wiswell's message resonated. American doctors have long associated the foreskin with infectious agents. Once his data and conclusions percolated into medical literature, some viewed the evidence in favor of circumcising to reduce the incidence of UTI as so conclusive that one Tulane urologist confidently wrote an article called "Neonatal Circumcision: An End to the Controversy?"[70]

This was premature. While scarcely as dangerous as carcinoma or as complex as HIV, UTI turns out to be a slippery condition. During the first year of life, UTI occurs more often in boys than in girls, though it is uncommon in either sex. One paper reporting incidence in a hospital in Israel noted that the median age for males diagnosed with UTI was sixteen days, whereas for females it was seven months. (The pediatricians hypothesized that ritual circumcision on the eighth day "may be a predisposing factor for UTI during the 12-day period following that procedure.") The disparity between male and female rates increases with age. By one year, UTIs become ten times more common in girls. Between twenty and fifty years of age, women's incidence of UTIs is fifty times greater than men's. Once a male is beyond infancy the disorder is rare, and the evidence is mixed about whether being circumcised makes any difference in susceptibility.[71]

The neonatal period is an appropriate focus of concern, because most infections in boys occur during the first six months of life. And premature birth creates special risks. "Urinary tract infection is much commoner in children than is widely believed," warned writers in the *British Medical Journal* in 1994. Still, the actual incidence is impossible to pin down, because the disease is often self-limiting and symptoms, if they appear at all, disappear without the child ever being diagnosed. "Although bacteriuria may be found in 1 to 2 per cent, asymptomatic children have a very high rate of spontaneous clearing of the bacteriuria and they seem to constitute a low-risk group," observed a noted Swedish urologist. In addition, many cases diagnosed as UTI may in fact have been something else. Signs and symptoms are nonspecific, typically beginning with fever. In boys the most common causes are anatomical problems that result in voiding disorders. An inability to completely empty the bladder makes it susceptible. In severe cases, high pressure within the bladder may force urine back up the ureters, damaging the kidneys.[72]

Where do these bacteria come from? A newborn has no natural bacterial flora. Shortly after birth, however, bacteria appear in the baby's intestinal tract, most often transmitted by the mother. These bacteria can be highly contagious, and they strike before babies have had time to develop immunity to them. Some hospital nurseries have reported dangerous outbreaks of infection.[73] A variety of organisms, including bacteria, viruses, fungi, and parasites, can enter the urethra or find another way into the bloodstream. Studies indicate that 85 percent of UTIs in males are caused by bacteria from the patient's own intestines. When a team of urologists examined the surgically removed foreskins of infants, they found that bacteria—in particular P-fimbriated *E. coli,* the culprit in most cases of UTI—colonized the inner mucosal surface of the prepuce. Still, the simple presence of these bacteria by itself produces no symptoms. Problems start when bacteria migrate through the urethra. Bacteria may infect the urethra, causing aperistalisis, or colonize the bladder, causing cystitis. Sometimes the same bacteria stick to renal tubular cells, provoking acute pyelonephritis. Circumcision prevents this chain of events because removing the foreskin removes the tissue on which the *E. coli* bacteria first adhere and propagate.[74]

In children whose urinary tract anatomy is normal, UTI is either self-limiting or easily treatable with antibiotic drugs, carrying little risk of kidney disease. Evidence suggests that the victims of recurring UTIs are not a random cross-section of the population. They seem to have a biological predisposition that makes them vulnerable to infection. Children born prematurely, according to one study of an inner-city population, showed an incidence of bacteriuria nine times greater than did term infants. Sometimes, when it goes undetected and untreated, pyelonephritis can threaten renal function. A study of renal disorders in Nigeria, for instance, showed that kidney disease accounted for 1.1 percent of Rivers State's total pediatric outpatient and hospital admissions. But the fuller health consequences of such infections are unclear. The American Academy of Pediatrics Task Force on Circumcision pointed out in 1999 that "the relationship between renal scar formation and renal function is not well defined, and the long-term clinical significance of renal scars remains to be demonstrated."[75]

Finally the issue of circumcision and UTI, like cancer and STDs, must be broken into a theoretical question—What does science tell us?—and a practical question—What should we do? We can combine these to ask: What should one do when the science is ambiguous?

Writing several years ago in the journal *Clinical Pediatrics*, J. B. Chessare, a physician interested in evidence-based medical practice, constructed a model decision tree for weighing the pros and cons of circumcision to prevent UTI. Based on a cross-section of medical literature, he estimated that the probability of a boy's contracting a UTI in the first year of life was 4.1 percent if he was uncircumcised and 0.2 percent if he was circumcised. For those who did become infected, he appraised the further, more serious risk of renal scarring at 7.5 percent. Turning to the risks of circumcision—bleeding, infection, and so forth—he figured the probability of minor complications to be 21.8 percent. (This is notably higher than ranges commonly reported in medical journals, which run between 0.19 percent to 10.0 percent.) Nonetheless, what is fascinating is Chessare's claim that the rate of minor complications from circumcision has no bearing on the decision to circumcise. Ranking all possible outcomes from worst (circumcision with UTI) to best (no circumcision, no UTI) and assigning each its own probability, he projected that the highest value would be achieved by not circumcising. According to his analysis, the rate of UTI in uncircumcised boys would have to reach 29 percent before the decision to do a preventive operation made sense.[76]

When in 1996 the Canadian Paediatric Society debated the costs and benefits of circumcision to prevent UTI, they turned to a thought experiment proposed several years earlier. The idea was to imagine a trial that enrolled 2,000 newborns, randomly circumcising half of them. Assuming a tenfold greater risk of UTI in the uncircumcised cohort—1.0 percent versus 0.1 percent—one would expect to see nine additional cases of UTI during the first year of life for every 1,000 infants not circumcised. Put in positive terms, 99.9 percent of circumcised boys and 99.0 percent of those left intact would not come down with UTI. But depending on the rate one applied, the surgery came with complications that could more than offset the lower risk of UTI. Assuming that postsurgical complications and UTI represent comparable health risks, the complication rate would have to be well below 1.0 percent to produce a benefit to one boy in a thousand. The Canadian pediatricians failed to see the wisdom in performing tens of thousands of operations to wring out such minute (and theoretical) benefits.[77]

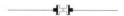

Much as people want a clear answer from medical science, the available evidence about circumcision is inconclusive. If we cannot pin down the effects on HIV susceptibility or infectivity (a basic distinction most published studies fail to recognize), how can we begin to weigh all the competing claims about everything from side effects to penile carcinoma? There is no Schroedinger equation for expressing how the influenza virus makes a person sick; there is no way for parents to predict whether circumcising their son will make him healthier.

A few clinical researchers have tried to draw together the different strands of investigation and to estimate an overall effect. One group built a model incorporating most published evidence of risks associated with being circumcised or uncircumcised. Using quality-adjusted years of survival as their measure, based on a life expectancy of 85 years, they figured that the average man circumcised at birth could expect to live 84.999 years, whereas his uncircumcised counterpart would live 84.71 years. A subsequent study that included more recent findings about UTI determined that, all things considered, being uncircumcised would shorten an average man's life by a total of fourteen hours. Statistically, the known pros and cons of circumcision cancel each other out.[78]

Indeed, the largest and most comprehensive examination of circumcision's overall long-term effects—based on a probability sample drawn from the National Health and Social Life Survey of 1,410 American men aged eighteen to fifty-nine years—is rich with ambiguity. "Circumcision status does not appear to lower the likelihood of contracting an STD," wrote Edward Laumann, the study's principal investigator. "Rather, the opposite pattern holds." But as one looked at more factors, the picture grew complicated. Gonorrhea, for instance, proved to be more common in uncircumcised men who had fewer lifetime sexual partners; as the average number of sex partners increased, however, gonorrhea was reported much more frequently in circumcised men. Sexual dysfunction, which bothered 45 percent of men in Laumann's sample, appeared not to be a function of circumcision status. With advancing age, though, "almost every dysfunction is slightly more common among men who have not been circumcised."[79]

While the medical variance between circumcised and uncircumcised men was negligible to slight, the same could not be said of the two groups' sex lives. "We find that circumcised men engage in a more elaborated set of sexual practices," Laumann wrote. Or, as the chic Internet e-zine *Salon* summarized the story, "It makes no health difference whether you're cut or not, but you'll get around more if you are." Essentially, the study concluded that on average, circumcised men engaged in heterosexual oral and anal sex and homosexual oral sex more commonly than their uncircumcised peers. Ironically, in light of the old theory that the foreskin encouraged masturbation, circumcised men were much more prone to masturbate. In the pages of the *Journal of the American Medical Association*, Laumann declined to speculate on these differences; but in subsequent interviews, he guessed that

> [t]here is possibility that circumcised penises are less sensitive because of the cutting of the head. So these men develop different ways of arousal and foreplay and also don't come as quickly; they are less likely to prematurely ejaculate. In the course of developing their sexual conduct people find these activities more appealing and pleasurable.

He added that the difference in rates of oral sex might have to do with self-consciousness on the part of uncircumcised men in a society where circumcision is the norm. "Their partner might associate an uncircumcised penis with bad hygiene—or that it's a smelly penis."[80]

Asked why people continue to circumcise their sons, Laumann replied:

> Mostly for cosmetic reasons. Parents say, "I want him to look like his dad and I don't want him to feel embarrassed in the locker room." The whole issue is a social issue, not a health or medical issue. People take tidbits of information and run with it. It's also a moneymaker. It costs about $250–$300 to perform a circumcision; and kids who have it have to stay in the hospital a little longer, which costs more.

Needless to say, those physicians for whom belief in the scientific validity of circumcision had long since hardened into faith remained defiant.[81]

SEVEN

Backlash

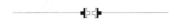

It cannot be ethical for a doctor to amputate normal tissue from a normal child.

—*John P. Warren et al.,* British Medical Journal *(1996)*

IN THE SPRING OF 1989, ACTIVISTS GATHERED ACROSS THE STREET FROM DISNEYLAND in Anaheim, California, to convene the First International Symposium on Circumcision. At the end of three days of presentations and discussion on topics ranging from "Circumcision as Child Abuse" to "Female Circumcision: Field Observations in Egypt," the attendees produced a policy statement that was after far-ranging debate adopted as the group's manifesto. "We recognize the inherent right of all human beings to an intact body," the declaration began.

> We recognize that the foreskin, clitoris and labia are normal, functional parts of the human body.
>
> Parents and/or guardians do not have the right to consent to the surgical removal or modification of their children's normal genitalia.
>
> Physicians and other health-care providers have a responsibility to refuse to remove or mutilate normal parts of the body.

Their statement went on to characterize those who had undergone circumcision, male and female, as "victims," and in scathing tones to "place the medical community on notice" for misleading the public, breaching medical ethics, and violating the United Nations Universal Declaration of Human Rights' injunction against torture and "cruel, inhuman or degrading treatment."[1]

The symposium was the consummation of a movement that had been gathering strength for more than a decade. It consisted of an assortment of physicians, medical professionals, gay rights activists, and others whose antipathy to genital cutting was almost religious in intensity.

At the center was a nurse named Marilyn Milos, whose life had been permanently changed when as a nursing student she witnessed her first circumcision. By that time she was already the mother of three sons, each circumcised on advice from her doctor, who, she said, "told me the surgery was a necessary health measure, that it didn't hurt, and that it took only a moment to perform . . . like cutting the umbilical cord."

On the fateful day, she joined her fellow nursing students in the hospital nursery where they found "a baby strapped spread-eagle to a plastic board on a counter top across the room. He was struggling against his restrains—tugging, whimpering, and then crying helplessly." Her natural instinct was to comfort the child. When the surgeon arrived, he suggested she put her finger into the baby's mouth to pacify him. But nothing had prepared her for what happened next.

> The silence was soon broken by a piercing scream—the baby's reaction to having his foreskin pinched and crushed as the doctor attached the clamp to his penis. The shriek intensified when the doctor inserted an instrument between the foreskin and the glans (head of the penis), tearing the two structures apart. (They are normally attached to each other during infancy so the foreskin can protect the sensitive glans from urine and feces.) The baby started shaking his head back and forth—the only part of his body free to move—as the doctor used another clamp to crush the foreskin lengthwise, which he then cut. . . . The baby began to gasp and choke, breathless from his shrill continuous screams. . . . My bottom lip began to quiver, tears filled my eyes and spilled over. I found my own sobs difficult to contain. . . . During the next stage of the surgery, the doctor crushed the foreskin against the circumcision instrument and then, finally, amputated it. The baby was limp, exhausted, spent.

Aghast as she was, Milos was astonished to hear the physician, his deep voice audible beneath the baby's screaming, casually remark, "There's no medical reason for doing this."[2]

This incident shocked and inspired Milos. Quietly at first, then with increasing boldness, she moved to alert the public to the evils of circumcision. She began to write and speak and distribute tracts. There was no mistaking her withering indictment of the medical profession, whose callous indifference to suffering and lofty pretensions of scientific authority struck her as hypocritical so long as doctors ignored the brutality of cutting infants' genitals. "After I saw my first infant circumcision," she recalled, "I began my work to stop the scream of babies, and suddenly men began to scream." In 1985, her agitation brought her to a crisis point when the California hospital that employed her fired her for, as she put it, "providing accurate information to parents." On reflection she realized that her dismissal was serendipitous, leaving her free to pursue her crusade full time. She lost no time in launching a vehicle for the campaign, establishing in the San Francisco Bay Area the National Organization of Circumcision Information Resource Centers (NOCIRC). This turned out to be the first national clearinghouse in the United States for information about circumcision. It advertised itself, on the Worldwide Web and elsewhere, as an organization "Dedicated to making a safer world [and] to securing the birthright of male and female children and babies to keep their sexual organs intact."[3]

At the heart of this effort was a belief in the sanctity of the body, coupled with moral indignation at those who, in Milos's words, fail "to respect the natural integrity of the male newborn's body. . . . Only by denying the existence of excruciating pain, perinatal encoding of the brain with violence, interruption of maternal-infant bonding, betrayal of sexual trust, the risks and effects of permanently altering normal genitalia, the right of human beings to sexually intact and functional bodies, and the right to individual religious freedoms can human beings continue this practice."[4]

In its first decade, NOCIRC expanded into a worldwide association of more than 90 centers. It quickly came to encompass a coalition of critics whose attacks on circumcision appeared throughout the 1980s. At the beginning of the decade, Edward Wallerstein, a retired industrial engineer and communications coordinator at New York City's Mount Sinai School of Medicine, published *Circumcision: An American Health Fallacy* (1980), a wide-ranging critique that sought to deflate the standard medical arguments for the procedure. Five years later, a nurse and alternative-child-rearing advocate, Rosemary Romberg, authored an emotional book, *Circumcision: The Painful Dilemma* (1985), concentrating on the violence circumcision visited on male infants and its possible psychological aftershocks which she strongly believed contributed to an increasingly violent American society. Then, in the mid-1980s, as NOCIRC's agitation increased around the United States and abroad, dozens of splinter groups devoted to various aspects of sexual surgery sprang into existence.

One of the most visible was the National Organization to Halt the Abuse and Routine Mutilation of Males (NOHARMM), a confederation of support groups from Alabama to Hawaii active in distributing educational materials, news releases, petitions, bumper stickers, decals, T-shirts, and videos.

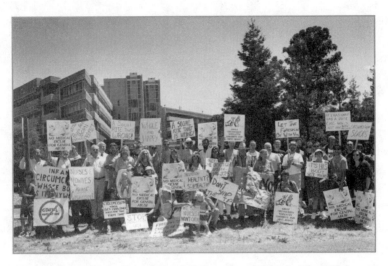

Demonstrators at Marin General Hospital, Greenbrae, California, July 1995. James Loewen, *Marilyn Milos personal collection*

By the late 1990s, NOCIRC and organizations that shared its basic outlook constituted a global movement. They relied on tried-and-true techniques of grassroots organization, holding small group meetings in apartments and churches, writing articles and letters to editors in local newspapers, bombarding opinion leaders with phone calls, faxes, and e-mail messages. Building alliances with medical associations, human rights groups, feminist organizations—virtually anyone who could help advance their agenda—the opponents of circumcision constructed a sophisticated network. At the same time, they also pieced together a new conceptual framework for circumcision, locating the issue within the larger legal and moral context of bioethics and human rights.

In structure, the arguments are simple. A 1996 letter published in the *British Medical Journal* from more than a dozen men who claimed injury from childhood circumcisions conveys the main points succinctly.

> The European charter for children in hospital states that every child must be protected from unnecessary medical treatment. The United Nations Convention on the Rights of the Child states that children have rights to self-determination, dignity, respect, integrity and non-interference and the right to make informed decisions. Unnecessary circumcision of boys violates these rights.

As for the medical profession, the writers conclude, "It cannot be ethical for a doctor to amputate normal tissue from a normal child."[5]

Even the uses of the amputated tissue were called into question. The notion of babies' foreskins being used to manufacture commercial products like cultured skin—even products designed to help patients with severe disorders—was anathema to the anticircumcision community. Upon learning that cancer researchers used foreskins as a source of interferon, one outraged writer approached the American Cancer Society demanding to know:

> How much does one infant foreskin sell for?
>
> How many have been sold?
>
> Who sells them? Doctors? Midwives? Mohels? Hospitals?
>
> Who buys them?
>
> Are there any "middle men," and if so, who are they?
>
> Are the foreskins sold "per foreskin" or by weight? (Do circumcisers have a financial incentive to cut off as much skin as possible?)
>
> Is a foreskin still marketable if it has been covered with or injected by an anesthetic? (Do circumcisers have a financial incentive not to use an anesthetic?)
>
> Are some types of foreskins more in demand than others? (White, Black, Latino, oriental [*sic*]?)[6]

This assault on medical research using foreskin tissues closely resembles attacks that Right to Life groups would mount on the use of fetal tissue, frozen embryos, and stem cells at the end of the twentieth century.

Eventually, activists managed to insert a provision in the United Nations International Covenant on Civil and Political Rights declaring that "slavery, forced labor, and traffic in persons includes the industry of a growing number of American medical hospitals and medical professionals colluding with scientific agencies *harvesting* neonatal foreskins for skin grafts, i.e., as compulsory organ donations."[7]

Appeals to human rights and concomitant efforts to enforce rights through the enactment of laws inform the tactics of organized opposition to male and female circumcision. It is therefore worthwhile to review their foundations.

For many centuries, Western medicine conformed, in theory if not in practice, to the ideals expounded by the Greek physician Hippocrates. The Hippocratic Oath, which gradually became a standard profession for new physicians, sets forth the principle of restraint: "I will use my power to help the sick to the best of my ability and judgment; I will abstain from harming or wronging any man by it." Better known, though, is an aphorism attributed to Hippocrates, compiled in the *Epidemics*: "As to diseases make a habit of two

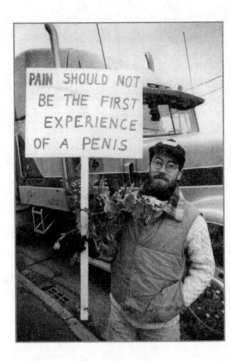

Opposition to cir-
cumcision comes
from a broad range
of activists.
James Loewen,
*Marilyn Milos per-
sonal collection*

things—to help, or at least, to do no harm" (Book 1, chapter 11). Since the
scalpel obviously produces immediate harm, surgeons have generally taken
Hippocrates to mean "don't do more harm than good."

Before World War II, medical ethics and the question of what rights people should enjoy with respect to their bodies were mostly discussed in terms
of the individual doctor-patient relationship. But in the wake of the war this
changed swiftly. Fiendish human experiments conducted by German medical
scientists were publicized as part of the Nuremberg war crimes trials, and four
Nazi doctors were hanged for crimes against humanity. During these trials, it
became obvious that no clear standard of ethical conduct existed for medicine
and medical research. The Nuremberg Code, drafted in 1947, was an international attempt to rectify this. By common agreement, the most important of
its ten points was the first: "The voluntary consent of the subject is essential."[8]

In the decades that followed, the United Nations, acutely sensitive to issues
involving power and exploitation, provided an international forum for increasingly explicit delineation of rights. That women and children were "entitled to special care and assistance" was a basic tenet of the Universal
Declaration of Human Rights (1948). Eleven years later, the General Assembly passed a nonbinding resolution called the Declaration of the Rights of the
Child (1959) that among other things sought to protect children from cruel

and abusive practices. It took another thirty years and the emergence of a postcolonial United Nations to produce a resolution called Implementation of the Convention on the Rights of the Child (1989), a document binding 176 nations to "protect the child from all forms of physical or mental violence, injury or abuse" and torture (Articles 19, 37, and 39).

In light of this imperative, did a routine neonatal procedure performed on most American males qualify as abuse or torture? NOCIRC and its fellow activists zealously insisted that it did. They flooded physicians and hospitals with letters and leaflets; and they took to the streets, demonstrating raucously at conventions of medical specialists to publicize their cause. In 1993, NO-HARMM picketed the annual meeting of the California Medical Association. Earlier, three nurses at St. Vincent Hospital in Santa Fe, New Mexico, had given the movement its first "conscientious objectors to circumcision" when they informed hospital administrators that they henceforth refused to assist in neonatal circumcisions. Another twenty nurses soon joined them. The public dispute between the nurses of St. Vincent and the medical establishment, widely televised on evening news shows and quickly made into a documentary film, exemplified a struggle that was becoming deeply politicized as circumcision advocates and opponents each claimed the moral high ground as its own.[9]

At heart, Milos did not view hers as a protest movement:

I'd like to make the point that we are not about "protest" as much as we are about human rights and truth. The demonstrations were a way to bring attention to the issue when the media were reluctant to cover this taboo subject. The history of circumcision in the West is not about differences of opinion. It is about the infiltration of genital mutilation of infants and children into Western medicine. I don't deny I am passionate about the issue, and it is because I was a mother first, before I saw a circumcision as a nursing student. It's been twenty years (this month) that I've been living with the screams of the baby in my ears—a sound I have never heard come out of the mouth of a human being, except during circumcision (and I have four children!). I am as chilled and disturbed by it today as I was twenty years ago, and I know that this is consistent with post traumatic stress.[10]

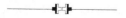

Many physicians felt themselves caught in the middle. Under growing pressure from anticircumcision forces and increasingly challenged by a patient population who turned out to be far more skeptical than their parents when it came to medical authority, physician groups faced a peculiar dilemma. What official position should they take on circumcision? Within large associations such as the American Academy of Pediatrics, the membership was deeply divided both in philosophy and custom. Other specialty societies—obstetricians, urologists, family practitioners, and so forth—grappled with circumcision, but the AAP's persistent effort to navigate a tortuous path through scientific evidence, received wisdom, and cultural and professional preferences best illustrates the profession's predicament.

Earlier we saw that the popularity of neonatal circumcision mirrored the rise of pediatric medicine, with its growing medicalization of birth and children's development. By the 1920s, in most modern American hospitals, after a mother gave birth a pediatrician was called to check the baby's health and, if the baby was a boy, circumcise him. Thus, at an early stage in the development of the specialty, circumcision became a trademark pediatric intervention, something of accepted benefit that the doctor could do beyond merely measuring and weighing the infant. As such, circumcision became an accepted part of American pediatric medical education and residency programs. For generations, no one imagined that this needed official sanction. Like most associations, the AAP defended the autonomy of its members and took a *laissez faire* approach toward standard procedures, letting individual practitioners decide what was right for their patients. By the early 1970s, however, new questions were surfacing about the efficacy of circumcision. Indeed, the AAP's Committee on Fetus and Newborn, in the process of publishing *Standards and Recommendations for Hospital Care of Newborn Infants* (1971), noted explicitly that "there are no valid medical indications for circumcision in the neonatal period."[11]

To silence its critics, the AAP at last appointed a task force to explore what official position if any the academy should adopt. When it was completed and published in *Pediatrics* in fall 1975, the task force report startled the medical community. Based on analysis of pertinent medical literature, the advisory panel reaffirmed the 1971 statement and declared that "a program of education to continuing good personal hygiene would offer all the advantages of routine circumcision without the attendant surgical risk. Therefore, circumcision of the male neonate cannot be considered an essential component of adequate total health care." Yet the report offered two crucial caveats. First, if the decision were made not to excise the foreskin, "the necessity for lifelong penile hygiene should be discussed with parents." Reading this warning, readers would reasonably infer that while it might not be absolutely essential, circumcision was probably a simple solution to an unpleasant problem. Hygiene, after all, with all its cultural connotations, had for many decades constituted the main rationale for neonatal circumcision. Critics immediately chided the AAP for fostering the myth that the foreskin needed more maintenance than other parts of the body.[12]

The second qualification compounded the confusion even further. Because "traditional, cultural, and religious factors play a role in the decision made by parents, pediatrician, obstetrician, or family practitioner on behalf of a son," the task force opined, "it is the responsibility of the physician to provide parents with factual and informative medical options. . . . The final decision is theirs, and should be based on true informed consent." In other words, though lacking a medical basis for operating, doctors should engage parents in discussion covering culture and religion to discover whether or not they wanted an unnecessary procedure. How such factors should be weighted, no one said—and if the surgery wasn't medically indicated, what precedents existed for cutting a normal child? Even if they had the time and inclination, few pediatricians had the command of history, tradition, and religion to engage parents in such a discussion. At best they were left to create informed consent based on their own experience. Far from obliging physicians to change their behavior, the earnestly ambiguous AAP task force report merely enabled them to justify their own preferences.[13]

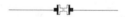

With such ambiguity emanating from its leadership, it is easy to see why, over the decades, AAP positions had little effect in the clinic. Restated in 1977 and 1983 and joined by the American College of Obstetrics and Gynecology, the policy lingered for a dozen years. During that period, however, the anticircumcision backlash intensified, as did the enthusiasm of a minority of pediatricians—newly convinced by a spate of published studies asserting that the procedure had notable preventive benefits—for waging a counterattack.[14]

In the meantime, the rising noise level attracted the attention of national broadcast media. In 1987, Phil Donahue, at that time the country's most popular television talk show impresario, devoted a full hour of "Donahue" to an encounter with five opponents of circumcision. These included Marilyn Milos and Dean Edell, a Jewish physician and father of five sons (three circumcised, two not) whose syndicated radio show boasted a national following of its own. Responding to a woman caller who defended circumcision because her husband, uncircumcised as an infant, suffered "infections" that finally resulted in his undergoing the procedure at age twenty-eight, Edell said, "A certain small percentage of men with foreskins will get disease of the foreskin, but you can't just remove everybody's. You can't pull everybody's teeth to avoid cavities, remove breast tissue from little girls so they won't get breast cancer." The show was both provocative and revealing. Above all, it showed that the lay audience was as perplexed by claims and counterclaims about circumcision's health benefits as they were opinionated about their own prejudices.[15]

A year later, ABC medical editor Timothy Johnson produced a segment of the network's "Nightline" in which Edell appeared together with a urologist, a pediatrician, and Benjamin Spock, the most celebrated baby doctor of the postwar generation. Introducing the subject, Johnson accurately summarized the problem. "The decision that parents must often quickly make," he said, "is increasingly complicated, and unfortunately, medical science cannot yet offer easy answers about risks versus benefits." Asked about his own views over the years, Dr. Spock, whose classic *Baby and Child Care* had sold more than 30 million copies, told viewers that although he had favored circumcision in the 1930s and 1940s, he'd since changed his mind.

> I'm against routine circumcision . . . if I had a baby boy now—I would love to have a baby boy—I certainly would not want him circumcised. And if parents ask me, I would lean in the direction of saying, "Leave his poor little penis alone." There's not enough proof that there's any danger from that. And therefore, let him be natural.

Others on the show expressed contrary opinions, especially a San Francisco urologist, Aaron Fink, who seized every chance he could to promote his forthcoming book, *Circumcision: A Parent's Decision for Life* (1988). But the skepticism of Drs. Spock and Lorraine Stern, a pediatrician from UCLA, made it clear, despite Fink's peremptory tone, that the medical evidence was at best equivocal.[16]

In March 1988, Fink briefly persuaded the California Medical Association to endorse a resolution affirming that circumcision was a valid public health intervention. And so the scene was set for the AAP Task Force on Circumcision Report of 1989.[17]

The task force was controversial from the start, not least because its chairman was Edgar J. Schoen. A member of the Department of Pediatrics at Kaiser Permanente Medical Center in Oakland, California, Schoen was a steadfast believer in circumcision. "Before the mid-1980s, the American standard of care included neonatal circumcision, a minor surgical procedure that promoted genital hygiene and prevented later penile cancer as well as cervical cancer in female sex partners," he flatly declared. He relished confrontation, going out of his way to ridicule those who disagreed with him. Two years before he was named to head the task force, Schoen published a bit of doggerel titled "Ode to the Circumcised Male" in the *American Journal of Diseases in Children*. Its purpose, he facetiously explained, was "to offer some solace to the generations of circumcised males who are now being told that they have undergone an unnecessary and deforming procedure, which may also have been brutal and psychologically traumatic."

> *We have a new topic to heat up your passions—the foreskin is currently top of the fashions.*
>
> *If you're the new son of a Berkeley professor, your genital skin will be greater, not lesser.*
>
> *For if you've been circ'ed or are Moslem or Jewish, you're outside the mode; you are old-ish, not new-ish.*
>
> *You have broken the latest society rules; you may never get into the finest of schools.*
>
> *Noncircumcised males are the 'genital chic'—if your foreskin is gone, you are now up the creek.*
>
> *It's a great work of art like the statue of Venus, if you're wearing a hat on the head of your penis. . . .* [18]

This smug tone and disdainful condescension carried over into Schoen's professional writings. Right or wrong, he was seldom open-minded and never uncertain.

Under Schoen's direction, the task force effectively reversed AAP's position. Conducting what appeared to be an exhaustive survey of the available medical literature, the group found much in favor of circumcision.

Properly performed newborn circumcision prevents phimosis, paraphimosis, and balanoposthitis and has been shown to decrease the incidence of cancer of the penis among U.S. men. It may result in a decreased incidence of urinary tract infection. . . . An increased incidence of cancer of the cervix has been found in sexual partners of uncircumcised men infected with human papillomavirus. Evidence concerning the association of sexually transmitted diseases and circumcision is conflicting.

Risks from the operation itself were glossed over: "newborn circumcision is a rapid and generally safe procedure when performed by an experienced operator." Pain—so often the theme of anticircumcision protest—was dismissed with the chilly observation, "Infants respond to the procedure with transient behavioral and physiologic changes." The task force concluded its report with an open-ended mantra: "Newborn circumcision has potential medical benefits and advantages as well as disadvantages and risks." Doctors thus were advised to spell out the benefits and risks (even though the report scarcely touched on the latter) chiefly to ensure that parents gave informed consent.[19]

When headlines in American newspapers and magazines trumpeted that the AAP now supported neonatal circumcision ("Pediatricians Find Medical Benefits to Circumcision" was how the *New York Times* reported the story), many of its members were appalled. "We have not reversed our position," insisted AAP president Donald W. Schiff. "We've changed it a bit, but it's really just a bit. . . . We're sort of opening the door a crack, so to speak, saying, 'We need to reexamine the issue and reidentify the data so that we know just what the facts are.' We don't have them all yet."[20]

While it is doubtful that the AAP's 1989 report influenced physicians' behavior any more than had previous statements, the furor surrounding its release exasperated the opponents of circumcision. "What's amazing to me," said Marilyn Milos, "is that they work so hard to sit squarely on both sides of the fence on this issue. They've given parents the responsibility to figure out what they (1) couldn't figure out, or (2) couldn't take a stand on." A lead story on Public Broadcasting Service's popular MacNeil-Lehrer News Hour, with experts lined up for and against the operation, perfectly captured the schism within the medical community, as well as the confusion on the part of parents as they tried to weigh competing epidemiological claims against their own prejudices and values.[21]

The issue continued to simmer. In 1996, confronted by a wave of new studies about the role of circumcision in preventing urinary tract infection and AIDS, the AAP once again appointed a Task Force on Circumcision. This panel of specialists and sub-specialists, headed by Carole Lannon, embarked on an exhaustive review of scientific evidence. After nearly three years, in March 1999, the task force published its "Circumcision Policy Statement." The group's ambivalence is clear from the abstract of their report:

Existing scientific evidence demonstrates potential medical benefits of newborn circumcision; however, these data are not sufficient to recommend rou-

tine neonatal circumcision. In circumstances in which there are potential benefits and risks, yet the procedure is not essential to the child's current well-
being, parents should determine what is in the best interest of the child. To
make an informed choice, parents of all male infants should be given accurate
and unbiased information and be provided the opportunity to discuss this decision. If a decision is made, procedural analgesia should be used.[22]

As in the past, the new policy was a compromise meant to reconcile the AAP's
hawks and doves. And like earlier statements, it concluded that while there was
no compelling medical reason to circumcise newborns, doctors and parents
might nonetheless conclude that it was in a child's best interests to be cut. But
on what basis? That he conform to his parents' idea of normal? That he look
like his father, or for that matter, his pediatrician?

News of the report was splashed across the popular press. The AAP generally was described as having reversed itself, withdrawing an important medical
sanction. But perhaps the most accurate comment came from veteran *New
York Times* health reporter Jane E. Brody, who wrote, "Those who have looked
to the nation's pediatric authorities for guidance are no doubt thoroughly
confused by now."[23]

Meanwhile, opposition within the physician community became increasingly assertive. In 1996 a Seattle physician named George Denniston organized Doctors Opposing Circumcision (DOC) to combat the vocal minority
of procircumcision physicians who, he claimed, "have been very effective, influential and far-reaching with their misinformation." Like so many other
activists, Denniston was a pamphleteer, having co-authored *Say No to Circumcision! 40 Compelling Reasons Why You Should Respect His Birthright and Keep
Your Son Whole* (1996).

For American physicians, the most credible word on medical science has
been peer-reviewed journal literature, with periodicals such as the *New England Journal of Medicine, Journal of the American Medical Association,* and *Archives
of Internal Medicine* at the top. In the view of some, though, mainstream medical journals harbored a strong bias in favor of circumcision, skewing the kinds
of studies they accepted for publication and leaving it to British and European
publications, little read in the United States, to fill out the picture. Robert Van
Howe, a pediatrician at the Marshfield Clinic in Wisconsin, grew increasingly
frustrated by "the inability of well-written credible studies relating to the prepuce to find a publishing home in mainstream American medical journals"
and finally resolved to launch an alternative review. The result was *Circumci-*

sion, a virtual journal first published on the Internet in June 1996. In the classic tradition of reform dissent, Van Howe and his colleagues waged a running battle with the mainstream, publishing letters to the editor that the *New England Journal of Medicine* and other publications had rejected, flaying procircumcision advocates for sloppy reasoning and poor experimental methods and subjecting their published papers to excruciating analysis. That this message resonated with certain younger doctors was clear from their responses. One intern at the University of California, San Diego, on pediatric rotation at the local Navy hospital, described his discomfiture at being required to discuss circumcision with new parents. "When we represent the medical literature to our patients, it is worse than giving them our personal bias," he wrote, "because it gives them a persuasion against which they have no defense. Therefore, I thank you for your lengthy criticism of the research that has supported the practice of male genital mutilation." In a postscript, the young doctor described his moral dilemma: "I felt like a low ranking Nazi soldier, lacking the moral fortitude to refuse doing what I know is wrong."[24]

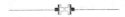

Although rhetoric casting routine neonatal circumcision as a matter of human rights and atrocity struck many physicians and others as undue hyperbole, it has turned out to be effective. On the level of principle, it linked male circumcision (which most Americans accepted as fairly benign) with female genital mutilation (which they considered cruel and repulsive). This connection increased the size of the activist network and also put proponents of male circumcision on the defensive by obliging them to explain exactly how cutting boys differed from cutting girls.

Even more significant, debate about the right to control one's own body tapped into a rich and more mature political controversy that had roiled America for two generations: the battle over abortion.

Abortion is seldom mentioned in relation to the anticircumcision movement, but the parallels are readily apparent. For example, a 1995 film entitled *Whose Body, Whose Rights? Examining the Ethics and the Human Rights of Infant Male Circumcision* was promoted as containing "uncensored footage of male genitalia and of actual infant circumcisions." The fascinating thing about the film is that in dramatizing its polemic against circumcision, it intermingles familiar idioms from both pro-life and pro-choice media. To begin with, the graphic display of circumcision reflects a technique frequently used by abortion opponents: bringing the camera into the operating room to evoke disgust by revealing the ugly reality of the procedure. In pro-life films the fetus is the main victim, whereas in the anticircumcision video *Whose Body, Whose Rights?* the victim seems to be the newborn. Yet as the video unfolds, our perspective on the victim changes. Interviews with circumcised men, who profess that the childhood operation permanently scarred them, and with women who feel betrayed by the medical profession or who suffered female genital mutilation point out that in the United States everyone suffers from circumcision's violence. A similar message—that abortion is a pervasive evil, damaging the moral fabric of any community that tolerates it—is a staple of pro-life discourse. With abortion, as with circumcision, partisans on both sides have endeavored to enlist scientific medicine to prove their cases. In the mid-1990s, when studies were published suggesting a link between abortion and elevated risk for breast cancer, right-to-life groups quickly seized on the new research, issuing dozens of press releases to broadcast the findings. Predictably enough, when a team of Danish researchers announced the results of a subsequent study that showed no meaningful connection, a leading pro-life organization rushed to print a piece headlined, "Flaws in the Danish Study."[25] And just as anticircumcision reformers have combed the world for horror stories of botched circumcisions—"Infant Bleeds to Death After Being Circumcised" (*Miami Herald*, 26 June 1993) and "Grand Jury to Probe Death of Baby After Circumcision" (*Des Moines Register*, 20 November 1982) are among dozens of headlines that circulate in pamphlets and tracts—opponents of abortion make ample use of the literature of atrocity. Visitors to a national prolife web site are offered dozens of links with such titles as "Los Angeles Woman Dies from Legal Abortion"; "Suzanne Logan's Story of How Abortion Paralyzed Her for Life"; and "Listing of People Kevorkian Has Helped Die."[26]

"Whatever affects us psychologically also affects us socially," writes Ronald Goldman in his book, *Circumcision: The Hidden Trauma*. Arguing that the violence of the operation disrupts the mother–son bond shortly after birth, Goldman asserts that American men on a massive scale are afflicted by post-traumatic stress disorder. The lingering aftershocks of circumcision, he writes, include low self-esteem, "avoidance of intimacy in male–female relationships" (which partly explains high divorce rates), disregard for women's sexuality, and most alarming, a pandemic of violence manifest in America's high rates of assault, rape, and murder. "Both rape and circumcision involve sexual organs and violence," he maintains. "Rape perpetrators' motivations and excessive, inappropriate anger reflect feelings of having been victimized themselves. It can be argued that in a broader sense, circumcision (what's done to children) could be considered to be a form of rape (they will do to society)."[27]

THE FORESKIN RESTORATION MOVEMENT

The most radical aspect of the popular backlash against circumcision is the foreskin restoration movement. Yet in historical perspective, we may think of it as a logical conclusion.

In the decades leading up to and following the turn of the twentieth century, the predominant Anglo-American sexual ethic revolved around constraint and control. In 1900, writing in *The Lancet*, E. Harding Freeland frankly acknowledged that "an argument against the universal adoption of circumcision [is] that the removal of the protective covering of the glans tends to dull the sensibility of that exquisitely sensitive structure and thereby diminishes sexual appetite and the pleasurable effects of coitus."[28] But for those who prized self-control over sensual indulgence, he continued, this should be cause for relief. Thirty-five years later, a physician with the improbable name of C. W. Cockshut explained why the foreskin should be removed, even though to do so is "against nature."

> That is exactly why it should be done. Nature intends that the adolescent male shall copulate as often and as promiscuously as possible, and to that end covers the sensitive glans so that it shall be ever ready to receive stimuli. Civilization, on the contrary, requires chastity, and the glans of the circumcised rapidly assume a leathery texture less sensitive than skin. Thus the adolescent has his attention drawn to his penis much less often.[29]

Sexual mores change, of course, and the closing decades of the twentieth century found a growing number of men more than willing to draw attention to the penis, and in the process to try to regain the sensitivity they felt had been stolen from them along with their foreskins.

Much of the impetus behind foreskin restoration is traceable to the Men's movement of the 1980s and 1990s, which, according to one advocate, has helped "men regain their inner losses in a society that has been very damaging to men and boys." Stirred by texts like poet Robert Bly's best-selling *Iron John* (1992), men who considered themselves victims of modern American culture organized groups such as Men's Rights, Inc., the National Men's Resource Center, and the Redwood Men's Center. Within these organizations, as they inventoried the diverse harms visited on modern men, certain subgroups fixed their attention on circumcision: "the universally shared wound of males in America."[30]

The gospel of uncircumcision has its prophet in Jim Bigelow, a Californian who describes himself as "college professor, therapist, clergyman and author." Bigelow traces the beginnings of the modern foreskin restoration movement to 1963, when a South African surgeon named Jack Penn performed plastic surgery on a middle-aged man who "had a circumcised penis and did not like it." When the patient asked him to operate to replace his lost prepuce, Penn thought it best to send him out for psychological testing. The results, however, "indicated a marked psychological disturbance due to his circumcision and that he was normal in every other way." Consequently, Penn offered surgical repair.

> The operation consisted of a "degloving" of the skin of the penis by means of a circumferential incision at the base of the penis with the skin pulled forward to cover the glans. A free graft was then applied to cover the entire new area from the tip of the prepuce to the base of the penis.

The outcome, in Penn's view, was an aesthetic success and "the patient was completely rehabilitated psychologically."[31]

There is no evidence that Penn's paper had much influence within the medical profession. Sporadically, journal articles appeared in which authors described techniques that could be used to stretch or graft skin to recreate a foreskin in the circumcised. One San Antonio physician, Donald Greer, made such procedures something of a subspecialty, performing by his own count thirty-five operations over several years. Still, through the 1970s and early 1980s, the rare man who wanted to reverse his circumcision usually met with skepticism or derision from physicians. There was a small underground network of doctors who would attempt foreskin restoration. But like abortion doctors, they seemed to work in the shadows.[32]

Because the medical establishment was, for the most part, the uncircumcision movement's foe, it seems inevitable that this movement would find expression outside the medical mainstream. This is precisely what happened in 1982, with the formation of Brothers United for Future Foreskins (BUFF). Less an organization than a grassroots affinity network, the kind of enterprise that draws together far-flung individuals who share a narrow preoccupation,

BUFF was the crucible for what its members dubbed "the Nonsurgical Fore-skin Restoration Method."

The existence of an organized movement to reverse circumcision attracted public attention in June 1987 on "Donahue" where, in a show devoted to circumcision, a guest named Richard Steiner extolled the virtues of foreskin restoration.

> STEINER: There's also a lot of sexual male dysfunction because of circumcision.
> DONAHUE: Richard Steiner was circumcised as a child and reversed the procedure in adulthood. They can do that now.
> STEINER: It can be done.
> DONAHUE: And you're a happier man now that you've—what do you call this? Decircumcision?
> STEINER: It's called a foreskin restoration procedure.

After showing his audience videotape of a circumcision, Donahue returned to Steiner, asking him to show his "arts and crafts." Steiner's account riveted the audience.

> I was sexually dysfunctional and it did cost me personally. It was a factor in my divorce, and I sought out a foreskin restoration procedure. I spent two years going from doctor to doctor, being thrown out of their offices, being laughed out of their offices and told I was crazy, I needed psychiatric help.

At last he found a doctor willing to operate.

> What the doctor does is he measures from the circumcision scar back up the shaft the same amount of skin, makes an incision all the way around it and then literally peels that skin down forward. And then he goes into the scrotal fat, he makes two horizontal incisions and creates a tunnel there. . . . The new foreskin [is] sewn into place, the front half is sewn into place for a period of anywhere from 10–16 weeks, so that blood veins and arteries can form and it becomes a healthy, living tissue. It's not just a flap of skin.

Once healed, the new foreskin changed Steiner's life. "Let me tell you," he declared, "any man, any woman, any rabbi, anyone who tells you there is not any difference in the sensitivity of an uncircumcised glans does not know what they're talking about."[33]

The show prompted a blizzard of mail. By breaking the story, it also conferred mainstream media legitimacy on a topic that formerly had been ignored or scorned as being of base prurient interest.

The Donahue audience that day included Jim Bigelow, to whom the show was a revelation. "Up to that point," he later wrote, "I did not know that anyone else felt as I did about being circumcised, and I certainly did not know there was any remedy." An instinctive organizer, Bigelow began to experiment with his own procedures for foreskin restoration. He quickly discovered ways to improve the techniques described in BUFF's leaflets and newsletters. By August 1991, after a few years of working with other groups, Bigelow founded his own association, which he called the UNCircumcising Information and Resources Center (UNCIRC).[34]

Several other groups coalesced around the same time. The most notable were the National Organization of Restoring Men (NORM) and the National Organization to Halt the Abuse and Routine Mutilation of Males. Both started in San Francisco where they found abundant sources of growth within the city's variegated gay culture. "The gay community was targeted first for this outreach," wrote R. Wayne Griffiths, because "gay men, in general, tended to be more open than their heterosexual counterparts about matters concerning sexuality in general and their genitals in particular." The groups, averaging a dozen or so attendees, met in their founders' apartments. They began to recruit others through classified advertisements in Bay Area newspapers. Within months, as its meetings swelled, RECAP (for Recover a Penis, the predecessor of NORM) began renting space on a monthly basis from the Metropolitan Community Church of San Francisco.

NORM's founders stated their aim "to create a safe place" where "men can share their concerns without fear of being ridiculed for a desire to be intact and whole again." They published a list of Governing Policies that included a strong rule of confidentiality, a prohibition on sexual activity at group meetings, and a statement that the group should not elect formal leaders but should set its agenda by consensus. The policies concluded by stating, "Due to the sense of woundedness of many of the men who participate in these groups and out of a sense of modesty, women will not be invited to attend the regular meetings."[35]

The foreskin restoration movement gained new currency during the Second International Symposium on Circumcision held in San Francisco in spring 1991. There Bigelow and Griffiths took the stage to present a slide show detailing the results of different methods of uncircumcision, including surgery and nonsurgical stretching.

Beyond everything else, opposition to circumcision and commitment to restoring the foreskin brought a certain type of isolated men together into a community. Leaders of this movement spoke of awakening men from a "circumcision coma." Tim Hammond, organizer of NOHARMM, expressed the sense of separation he had experienced.

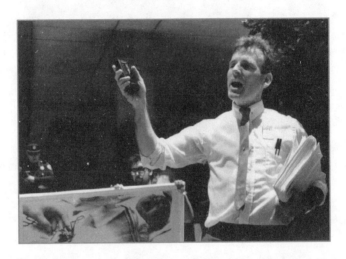

Tim Hammond, founder and director of National Organization to Halt the Routine Mutilation of Males (NOHARMM) demonstrating at a meeting of the California Medical Association.
James Loewen, *Marilyn Milos personal collection*

Awareness that this was done to you is something that a lot of circumcised guys more or less stumble upon. If he reads enough, he eventually learns that this circumcision was not only unnecessary, but deprived him of fully functioning genitalia. This widespread ignorance before such an awareness occurs is a kind of mental circumcision. Later, when he gets the message that people are uncomfortable talking about it, and he is treated like it's not important or that he shouldn't question it, a man becomes aware of being cut off from society, and then a deeper circumcision of the soul sets in.[36]

There is irony in Hammond's choice of words. Whereas St. Paul's "circumcision of the heart" metaphorically included an uncircumcised Gentile in the community of the Christian faithful, Hammond's "circumcision of the soul" expresses a profound sense of alienation.

Men who embarked on the painstaking course of foreskin restoration often described their decision as a quest for wholeness. They frequently compared foreskin restoration to the familiar use of plastic surgery to reconstruct women's breasts after cancer surgery. To those who dismissed this comparison, Jim Bigelow wrote: "We're just not accustomed, as yet, to thinking men have such feelings and needs, but they do." In support of this point, Bigelow recounted an episode from the late 1980s when he was teaching a sex therapy class in a small college. As part of the course, he individually interviewed fifteen male students, ranging in age from twenties to midforties, to find out how they felt about being circumcised. To his dismay, none voiced any negative feelings. A year and a half later, though, one of same men showed up in the same course and, when Bigelow reported his findings from the earlier interviews, asked for permission to address the class. The man, now twenty-four, said that he had recently married, and that owing to their strong religious beliefs he and his wife had entered marriage as virgins. What bothered him, however, was that "he had become keenly aware that his new wife brought to him a fresh, unaltered body just as God had designed it. While he, on the other hand, had an altered, disfigured body to offer her."[37]

Whether or not the men attracted to foreskin restoration have other reasons for feeling physically defective, it is clear that to most of them the penis is the source of a negative self-image that goes far beyond sexuality. Like victims of child abuse and rape, they voice feelings of powerlessness, vulnerability, and rage. The uncircumcision community aggressively encourages first-person narratives, and in hundreds of booklets, newsletters, and tracts, along with Internet bulletin boards and user groups, one encounters torrents of anger. "I was circumcised when I was five—seventy years ago," reported one man. "I felt rage then and I still feel rage now." Another said, "I think I could have accepted a deformity that was an accident of nature, but I can't accept that someone *did* that to me." Some men turned their anger outward. "Anger is a pallid euphemism for what I felt. More accurate would be overwhelming fury, rage, and desire for vengeance, desire to torture, maim, and utterly destroy any human being who ever had anything to do with performing, ordering, or requesting circumcision."[38]

Some men, aided by therapists, believe that they relive the pain and trauma of having been circumcised in infancy. One patient, under hypnosis, described his experience in these terms.

I don't know what's going on. I hear babies crying and I'm crying too. I don't know why. Oh! They are pulling on my penis and I'm feeling some pain. It hurts there; I'm not sure why. There's a white robe; it's a doctor. They are holding my legs down, and my back is arched. They are cutting my penis and it hurts. It hurts! I feel my penis being pulled. I feel sharp points there.[39]

For some men, circumcision exacerbates their sense of sexual anxiety, with a feeling that their genitalia are misshapen or inadequate. Indeed, much has been made of circumcision's effect on body image. "Cosmetics become a problem when the body image becomes involved," observed one team of sex researchers who interviewed men who had been circumcised as adults, "and may affect the entire sense of well-being, work capability included, as well as heterosexual bonding and family life."[40] The few studies that have attempted to gauge men's attitudes toward their own circumcision status suggest that once they understand the issue, uncircumcised men tend to be happier with their state than those who were cut in infancy. A 1996 study of 546 men sponsored by the anticircumcision group NOHARMM enumerated several physical consequences that respondents attributed to circumcision: scarring, "insufficient penile skin for comfortable erection," curvature of the erect penis, discomfort and bleeding during sexual activity. Of those who responded, 61 percent claimed that circumcision resulted in some sexual dysfunction, chiefly problems achieving erection and orgasm. Perhaps these feelings have special resonance in America owing to the common preoccupation with penis size as a measure of virility.[41]

The seamier reaches of the Internet and the back pages of men's magazines are filled with advertisements for gimmicks guaranteed to increase the size of the male organ. One web site at *http://www.surgeon.org/penis.html* features dozens of nonsurgical devices with such names as Dr. Kaplan's Penis Enlargement Vacuum Pump and The Circle Device–Penis Stretcher. [42]

Exploiting the same market, physicians offer a variety of surgeries and implants, at prices running from $2,000 to $10,000. Penile enlargement surgery, for example, involves release of the suspensory ligament connecting the penis to the pubic bone. This allows the surgeon access to the internal part of the penis, behind the patient's skin. The exposed erectile tissue is covered by a skin graft. According to a urologist who specializes in penile enlargement:

Well-motivated patients who follow post-operative instructions have achieved penis length gains up to 2 inches with the average increasing penis length about 1 inch. Men with prominent suprapubic fat pads will gain extra penis length. For example, if they have a 2-inch thick fat pad and 1½ is liposuctionable, their total gain will be 1½ inches plus whatever is gained by resecting the penile suspensory ligament.

In addition to lengthening the penis, surgeons also offer procedures to increase the organ's girth, either by harvesting fat cells from a man's lower abdomen or buttocks and transplanting them between the skin and erectile tissue of the penis or by inserting silicone strips. These are essentially cosmetic surgical procedures, using the same techniques and same materials (e.g., silicone) for female breast augmentation.[43]

In many respects, the process of foreskin reconstruction—so-called skin expansion—advocated by UNCIRC and similar groups shares the objective of augmenting the penis. "Visible skin over the glans is the goal of foreskin restoration," according to Bigelow. But the movement is explicitly nonmedical; that is, skin expansion is advertised as the prerogative of laymen, not doctors. As such, it combines elements of folk medicine and tribalism. Bigelow reminds his readers, "some of the first men who began to 'stretch' a new foreskin were impressed by customs of certain indigenous peoples, [and] some of the articles in prestigious medical journals also began by noting the distended earlobes and lips among these same peoples."[44]

Applying age-old principles of skin expansion, members of the foreskin restoration movement invented and constantly refined techniques for stretching out what remnants of a foreskin a circumcised man has left until, after some months, the skin is loose enough to pull over the end of the glans. The UNCIRC program basically employs surgical tape cut into various shapes or rings that men attach to the skin at the base of the penis, creating just enough tension to gradually stretch it. Some men attach small weights (lead fishing sinkers are suggested) to gradually protract an ersatz foreskin even further over the penis. In fact there is a thriving cottage industry in medical contraptions designed to hasten skin expansion. One device called the Tugger, formerly marketed as the Penis Uncircumcising Device (PUD), is a system of weights and elastic bands that retails for $115 plus shipping and handling; but most of the devices men use are homemade. The process of innovation, of discussing the progress of one's restoration and comparing one method to another, is an important part of the movement's shared culture.

The earliest expansion devices, worn by BUFF members in the early 1980s, were bizarre contraptions.

First, the individual either applied a tape "splint" to the exterior of his burgeoning foreskin or wore a hollow, spool-like device within his foreskin which
was stretched out and taped around and to the spool. . . . He then attached one
end of an elastic strap to the tip of the tape splint or of the protruding spool.
Next, he stretched the elastic strap and either attached the other end to a garter

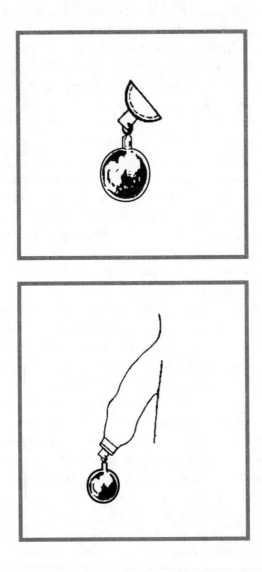

Sketch of a ball-bearing device used for foreskin
restoration. From Jim Bigelow, *The Joy of Uncircumcising!*
(2d ed., 1995).

worn below the knee of one leg or he pulled his penis, with the strap attached, backward between his scrotum and one leg. He then attached the other end of the stretched strap to the back of a garter belt worn at the waist.[45]

The process can take between three and five years. The aesthetic satisfaction men derive from gaining a foreskin, they claim, is less important than the increased sensitivity of the glans and mucous tissue. Bigelow writes that as the new foreskin is stretched over the glans, the skin changes texture and color. "Not only does the glans regain sensitivity, the mucous tissue which is typically between the glans and the circumcision scar also becomes much more responsive."[46]

The process and paraphernalia surrounding foreskin restoration amount to a secret ritual. Bigelow captures the idea:

At UNCIRC, we hear from doctors, ministers, schoolteachers, computer engineers, construction workers, truck drivers, etc., etc. You can just imagine the social situations these men are in and the thoughts that sometimes pop into their heads. Imagine, for instance, being a minister in the pulpit with your vestments on and suddenly realizing just what some of your congregation would think if they only knew that, at that very moment, you were wearing tape on your penis and restoring your foreskin! Some men find themselves chuckling right out loud. Far from the dread of discovery, which after all is quite controllable, many men report a little rush of delight and satisfaction as they realize once again that they are doing something for themselves at a very personal and private level and that they've got a little secret which they are keeping from most of the world.[47]

EIGHT

Female Circumcision

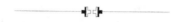

*The operation of circumcision in girls consists in the bloody amputation
and extirpation of the clitoris, as well as its prepuce, and in the amputation of the labia minora and the entrance of the vagina.*

—H. Ploss, Das Weib in Natur- und Voelkerkunde *(1887)*

THE MOST RECENT CHAPTER IN THE ANCIENT SAGA OF FEMALE CIRCUMCISION MAY
be said to have begun in 1994 when a seventeen-year-old Muslim woman
named Fauziya Kassindja arrived at Newark International Airport from the
Republic of Togo. She was traveling with a false passport, and when she arrived desperately approached immigration authorities with a plea for asylum.
Her reason: if she were sent back to West Africa, Kassindja claimed, she would
be forced to submit to ritual surgery on her genitals. Adding insult to injury,
this was to be preparation for an arranged marriage to a much older man who
already had three wives. Immigration officials, unimpressed with her story,
threw her into the Esmoor detention center in Elizabeth, New Jersey, where
at the hands of guards and keepers she endured a series of stark, humiliating
cruelties. There, and later in a similar facility in Pennsylvania, she languished
for two years while her appeal worked its way through the Immigration and
Naturalization Service (INS) bureaucracy. In the meantime, however, the news
of her ordeal spread, calling fresh attention to the plight of millions of women
and girls around the world who quietly endured various genital cutting procedures known as female circumcision.

From the day it was first reported in the *New York Times*, the story stirred waves of popular reaction on radio and television talk shows, in letters to newspaper editors and editorials. *Times* columnist A. M. Rosenthal, in a typical broadside, decried a "torture so hideous that most of humanity does not even want to think about it." He called on President Bill Clinton to endorse a three-point plan, including designating $100 million of the American foreign aid budget for local campaigns against ritual mutilation; giving more aid to countries that actively work to eradicate female genital mutilation "and less, or nothing" to those that don't; and making the issue a top priority for American delegations to the United Nations. This was the least that should be done to curtail procedures whose "short-term results include tetanus, septicemia, hemorrhages, cuts in the urethra, bladder, vaginal walls and anal sphincter. Long-term: chronic uterine infection, massive scars that can hinder walking for life, fistula formation, hugely increased agony and danger during childbirth, and early deaths."[1]

Kassindja's first hearing before immigration judge Donald V. Ferlise proved a disaster. Poorly represented by inexperienced, unprepared lawyers, her story failed to convince the judge. "I have taken into account the lack of rationality, the lack of internal consistency and the lack of inherent persuasiveness in her testimony," he said, "and have determined that this alien is not credible." Fortunately, the case attracted the attention of Karen Musalo, an experienced attorney who headed the International Human Rights Clinic at American University, Washington College of Law. Professor Musalo agreed to handle the appeal pro bono.[2]

Finally, in June 1996, the Board of Immigration Appeals granted Kassindja political asylum and in the process established fear of female genital mutilation as legitimate grounds for granting asylum. Thus female circumcision joined the previously accepted categories of persecution: race, nationality, religion, political views, and membership in a social group. In principle, the board ruled that Kassindja's Tchamba-Kunsuntu tribe persecuted women when it practiced ritual genital surgery. "Women have little legal recourse and may face threats to their freedom, threats or acts of physical violence, or social ostracization [*sic*] for refusing to undergo this harmful traditional practice," the ruling said.[3]

To most observers in the industrialized world and to Western media, female circumcision has seemed a barbaric maiming of girls' bodies. Indeed, in the late 1990s, the issue was everywhere in the media. The internationally famous fashion model Iman revealed that she had been permanently scarred by the ritual, and Waris Dirie, another fashion model who was born in Somalia and suffered an agonizing mutilation at age five, was appointed special ambassador to the United Nations to lead a crusade against ritualized female circumcision. Partly because of its harrowing account of her ordeal—"I remember thinking, after they tied me down on my back flat and left there completely hopeless, in agony, Why?"—Dirie's memoir, *Desert Flower*, became a best-seller in Europe. With tolerance waning, in February 1999, a French court sentenced an African woman to eight years in prison for cutting the genitals of forty-eight girls, all under the age of ten. The harshness of the sentence was clearly a message to the nation's large African immigrant population that mutilation would not be tolerated in modern France.[4]

Beneath the surface, however, to some reporters and scholars the picture was more complicated than it first appeared. One American reporter, exploring practices on the Ivory Coast, discovered that ritual surgery is deeply woven into the texture of family and cultural life. "It is part of a girl's dreams of womanhood, a father's desire to show off with a big party and a family's way of proving its conformity to social convention." In short, the traditions that supported genital cutting were quite similar to the values and ideals that sustained male circumcision in the same tribal societies. Female circumcision could not be described as a qualitatively different practice, ethnographer Felix Bryk observed in the 1930s, since it contained "the same motives, measure, and manners [as male circumcision] translated, like a print, in the service of the same idea, both erotic and social."[5]

Bryk's view remains controversial. Proponents of male circumcision contend that ritual cutting of girls is not circumcision at all but barbaric mutilation, usually carried out by people untrained in medicine: barbers, shamans, midwives, virtually anyone with a razor or a knife. While it is most common among Muslims, dozens of African, Middle Eastern, and Asian peoples routinely practice some form of female genital cutting, usually on young girls. The World Health Organization estimates that the global impact of these practices constitutes a serious public health crisis. As many as 2 million girls a year are subjected to some form of cutting, adding to a worldwide count of 130 million women and girls. Egypt, Ethiopia, Kenya, Nigeria, Somalia, and Sudan account for about three quarters of all cases. In some of these countries, more than 90 percent of the female population has been cut.

The nature of the operations varies widely. As with male circumcision in tribal settings, pain is integral to the ritual. In modern times, the operation is usually done without anesthetic. In past eras, there are reports of extraordinary measures to intensify the pain. One German explorer in Africa in the seven-

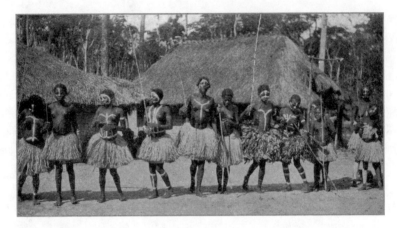

A group of Banta (Zaire) girls shortly before ritual cutting in the early 1930s.
From A. M. Vergiat, *Les Rites Secrets des primitifs de l'Oubangui* (1936).

teenth century horrified his readers by writing, "The girls also have their special circumcision; for when they have reached their tenth or eleventh year,
they insert a stick, to which they have attached ants, into their genitories, to
bite away the flesh, indeed, in order that all the more be bitten away, they
sometimes add fresh ants."[6]

At one extreme, in certain areas along the Indonesian archipelago, the local midwife or on occasion the infant's father scratches a girl's labia majora
with a sharp tool. No tissue is removed. Indonesians describe the operation as
kaanggui nepteppi sarat—merely the fulfillment of a ritual formality. In most
places, though, the surgery is invasive. The classical Muslim author al-
Mawardi, for example, limited it to "cutting off the skin in the shape of a ker-
nel located above the genitalia. One must cut the protruding epidermis
without performing a complete ablation." Yet there is little evidence that
midwives and other circumcisers bother with such fine distinctions. In much
of Egypt, female circumcision means removal of the clitoris, along with portions of the external labial tissue around the opening of the vagina.

Taking the whole process one step further, some African communities follow the ritual cutting of the clitoris and labia by sewing up the genitalia to
close off the vagina, leaving a small opening for the passage of urine and menstrual blood. This procedure is called infibulation, and its purpose is to make
sexual intercourse impossible until the girl is married. Since the sutured labial
tissue grows together over the years like a skin graft, significant surgery is necessary to reopen the vaginal passage. In some tribes, in Somalia, for example,
before the husband takes his bride, village women make an incision to open

her vagina and insert a phallus made of wood or clay, supposedly the shape and size of the husband's organ. This object may be left in place for days or weeks to prepare the bride for sexual union and, not incidentally, to prevent the wounded tissue from adhering and beginning to grow back together.

Jacques Lantier, a French doctor who traveled through Somalia in the early 1970s, attended such a ceremony and described it in grisly detail. The elderly woman who performed the procedure began by separating the girl's labia majora and labia minora and attaching them

> with large thorns onto the flesh of each thigh. With her kitchen knife the woman then pierces and slices open the hood of the clitoris and then begins to cut it out. While another woman wipes off the blood with a rag, the operator digs with her fingernail a hole the length of the clitoris to detach and pull out that organ. The little girl screams in extreme pain, but no one pays the slightest attention.

The circumciser excises the clitoris with her knife,

> then lifts up the skin that is left with her thumb and index finger to remove the remaining flesh. She then digs a deep hole amidst the gushing blood. The neighbor women who take part in the operation then plunge their fingers into the bloody hole to verify that every remnant of the clitoris is removed.[7]

Afterward, the vulva is sewn up with silk or catgut sutures. On the bride's wedding night, assured of his wife's virginity, the husband is supposed to cut the stitches with a knife before consummating the marriage. In some tribes, a woman is resewn if her husband travels for an extended time, or if she is divorced.[8]

The side effects vary. At the time of the operation, the greatest risks are hemorrhage and shock, which claim unknown numbers of victims each year. And while most girls survive, many experience acute or chronic disorder related to the surgery. Among the most common are clitoral cysts, labial adhesions, recurrent urinary tract infections, renal scarring and kidney dysfunction, sterility, and, as intended, loss of sexual feeling.

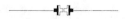

In the world of Islam, female circumcision has long been acknowledged as a rightful counterpart to male circumcision. Indeed, Islamic medicine, as early as the tenth century, presumed that male and female sexual organs were essentially alike. Al-Kunna al-Maliki told the early faithful that the vagina "possesses prolongations of skin called the lips," and that these are "the analogue of the prepuce in men," whose main function is to protect the organs from blasts of cold air.[9] Muslim female circumcision fascinated the illustrious Victorian British explorer Sir Richard Burton. "This rite is supposed by Moslems to have been invented by Sarah," he wrote, "who so mutilated Hagar for jealousy and was afterwards ordered by Allah to have herself circumcised at the same time as Abraham." He thought that it was the mirror image of male circumcision, "evening the sensitivities of the genitories by reducing it equally in both sexes." An uncircumcised woman would experience orgasm sooner and more frequently than her circumcised male partner, resulting in sexual disequilibrium.[10]

The chief sources of Muslim law and religious authority are the Koran, the *Sunnah* (the "path" marked by the Prophet Mohammed's words and deeds), and more recently the fatwas, opinions and teachings of Muslim religious scholars. The Koran itself is silent about female, as well as male, circumcision.

Yet the sayings of Mohammed, promulgated and interpreted by later scholars, do mention the practice, albeit ambiguously. Most commonly cited is a brief dialogue between the Prophet and a woman named Um Habibah, who was reputedly a circumciser of female slaves. Upon encountering her, Mohammed asked Um Habibah whether she continued to practice her profession. She said that she did, but that she would give it up if the Prophet disapproved. Far from objecting, he not only told her it was allowed, he also demonstrated the correct way to do the operation. "Come closer so I can teach you," he says in one version. "If you cut, do not overdo it, because it brings more radiance to the face and is more pleasant for the husband." Elsewhere, Mohammed is supposed to have recommended circumcision as a *sunnah* for men, meaning that it conformed to the right path, and a *makrumah* for women, suggesting that it was an estimable act, and to have stipulated that "if both circumcised parts meet or if they touch each other, it is necessary to wash before prayer." Still, the authenticity of these sayings is so dubious that even supporters of female circumcision give them little credence. According to Sheik Abbas, rector of the Muslim Institute at the Mosque of Paris: "There is no existing religious Islamic text of value to be considered in favour of female circumcision, as proven by the fact that this practice is totally nonexistent in most of the Islamic countries. And if unfortunately some people keep practicing excision, to the great prejudice of women, it is probably due to customs practised prior to the conversion of the people to Islam."[11]

It is rare to find any Muslim who questions male circumcision. Among clerics and scholars, however, female circumcision remains a source of intellectual puzzlement. The consensus seems to be that even if not explicitly commanded by the Prophet, it is nonetheless good, mainly because it curbs a woman's sexual desire and thus safeguards her morality. This was the reasoning of Cairo's influential Great Sheikh of Al-Azhar who, in 1981, warned parents to ignore the anticircumcision opinions of physicians and scientists on the grounds that medical science changes, whereas religious truth is constant and immutable. Parents, he warned, are the ones responsible for the moral welfare of their daughters. Alternatively, however, some Muslim scholars have argued that removing the hood of the clitoris would make a woman more sensitive during sexual intercourse, thus more likely to please her husband.[12]

Faced with growing international pressure, particularly from the World Health Organization, the conservative Islamic press has published dozens of articles that lay out a rationale for female circumcision. One doctor, Hamid al-Ghawabi, wrote that removing the clitoris and labia minora is essential to good hygiene, the only sure way to eliminate unpleasant odors in women. If it also happened to suppress sexual appetite, this was desirable as well. As men grow older, al-Ghawabi reasoned, their sex drive flags. A circumcised wife would be better suited to an aging man's needs than a woman so demanding that the husband could become embarrassed trying to satisfy her, and could risk using dangerous drugs to improve his potency. Others asserted that uncircumcised women risked nymphomania, clitoral swelling that could drive them to masturbation or lesbian activity, and even increased risk for vaginal cancer. According to its proponents, female circumcision eliminates a major source of excitability in girls and women and prevents them from "getting a yellow face," a sure sign of nervous anxiety.[13]

Regardless of theory, in the communities practicing it female circumcision expresses important social meanings. In the Egyptian countryside, the matron or midwife who typically performs the operation also provides a certificate of circumcision that the bride presents to her prospective husband before marriage. To remain uncut is to risk becoming an outcast. A Muslim woman named Nawal el-Saadawi, who had suffered from infibulation, explained the cultural power of genital mutilation this way:

> The importance given to virginity and an intact hymen in these societies is the reason why female circumcision still remains a very widespread practice . . . . Behind circumcision lies the belief that, by removing parts of girls' external genital organs, sexual desire is minimized. This permits a female who has reached the dangerous age of puberty and adolescence to protect her virginity, and therefore her honor, with greater ease. Chastity was imposed on male attendants in the female harem by castration which turned them into inoffensive eunuchs. Similarly female circumcision is meant to preserve the chastity of young girls by reducing their desire for sexual intercourse.[14]

Until the 1970s, the internal debate within Islam about female circumcision attracted little notice in the United States and Europe. Gradually, as the result of efforts by African activists and medical workers, including American missionaries and Peace Corps volunteers, a fuller picture of the nature and extent of ritual surgery began to emerge. Even so, there was no focused response until 1979, when an international health conference in Khartoum turned the spotlight on the health consequences for women and children of rituals and tribal practices in developing nations. This not only broke the silence; in an era of rising feminism, it also transformed female circumcision into a signal question of human rights.[15]

Female genital mutilation, so repulsive to Anglo-European sensibilities and to progressive Africans and Middle Easterners, became an important symbol in the larger war for women's and children's rights and improvements in reproductive health.[16] On the part of activists, the shift in nomenclature from *female circumcision* to *genital mutilation* was a wise move. People who respected individual cultural traditions might defend ancient ritual practices on grounds of cultural integrity, but virtually no one would try to defend mutilation. (Indeed, Islamic proponents of female circumcision typically argued that the cutting should only be done by experienced operators, and that the surgery should spare the clitoris.) Yet because the issue was so sensitive, it was not until 1994 that the term *female genital mutilation* found its way into international discourse. That year, in the wake of a CNN broadcast of a film showing the brutal circumcision of a ten-year-old girl by an unskilled circumciser, an International Conference on Population and Development in Cairo denounced such cutting as a fundamental violation of human rights. It called on governments to "prohibit and urgently stop the practice . . . wherever it exists." The chorus of opposition grew louder the next year at the Fourth World Conference on Women in Beijing, where the platform explicitly cited genital mutilation as a danger to women's reproductive well-being and a violation of their rights. With African women taking the lead, the final document strongly urged countries to pass and enforce strict laws "against the perpetrators of practices and acts of violence against women, such as female genital mutilation."[17]

Against this backdrop, in the early summer of 1997, Egyptian judge Abdul Aziz Hamade produced a shock of outrage that reverberated throughout the United States and Europe. Over the past year, he announced, his court had carefully deliberated the question of female circumcision and as a consequence had decided to strike down the Egyptian government's regulations banning surgery on girls' and women's genitals. Judge Hamade insisted that his ruling wasn't rooted in religion, sanctioning female circumcision within the context of Islam. It was, he maintained, purely a matter of proper medical prerogative. "Doctors' right to perform their profession according to the law— which allows them to do surgery—cannot be restricted by ministerial decree."[18]

The Egyptian court's ruling ignited a controversy that had smoldered for more than a decade. Egypt had been the target of a vigorous campaign orchestrated by human rights advocates and women's groups bent on outlawing female genital mutilation. Armed with surveys indicating that perhaps 80 percent of Egyptian women had suffered some form of cutting, in July 1996 they successfully pressured the Health Ministry to issue a regulation that prohibited ritual surgery on female genitals in licensed medical facilities, mainly state and private clinics.

But their moment of triumph was brief. Denouncing the ban as a departure from Islam, conservative religious leaders waged an aggressive campaign to overthrow it. Although the administrative elements of government had grown increasingly secular, the conservative Egyptian judiciary proved sympathetic to old-fashioned religious arguments, including one cleric's assertion that women "who are not circumcised get AIDS easily."

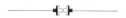

Ritual cutting of females is perhaps as old as male circumcision and its origins and early meanings are equally cryptic. Early in the first century A.D., the Greek historian Strabo found evidence that the ancient Egyptians circumcised females as well as males. A fourth-century papyrus from St. Ambrosius of Milan noted: "The Egyptians circumcise their males at their fourteenth year, and the women are said to be circumcised the same year because from that time the passion of sex begins to burn and monthly period of women begins." But no wall carvings memorialize the female ritual. A number of authors in antiquity explained female circumcision as an aesthetic measure—something to correct or improve the appearance of female genitalia, especially in cases where the labia minora seemed unnaturally large. Against those who have criticized female circumcision as an invention of Islam, one Muslim scholar has argued that, beginning in the first century A.D., "it was Judaic mythical beliefs and later practices, combined with Christian compromises, that helped spread the practice through many cultures." In truth, however, no one knows the early history.[19]

What seems evident is that across different cultures the most basic rationale for female circumcision stems from the simple fact that for most of history, women were thought to have essentially the same genitalia as men, the only real difference being, in the words of one fourth-century commentator, that "theirs are inside the body and not outside it."[20] Through the Renaissance, anatomists depicted the labia as the vagina's foreskin. And male-oriented nomenclature persists down to this day. For example, Frank Netter's *Atlas of Human Anatomy* labels the tissue covering the clitoris "prepuce of clitoris," and the organ itself "glans of clitoris."[21]

The utility of the operation, beyond its obvious dulling of women's sexual sensations, remained a subject of speculation among ethnographers. In the late nineteenth and early twentieth centuries, many students of African cultures surmised that "the operation was performed only to lessen the extraordinarily active sexual instinct of women among the African tribes." Some agreed with the early Danish traveler Carsten Niebuhr that the motive was cleanliness, "that thereafter the women may be able the more conveniently to wash themselves." Others conjectured that the reasons must have been cosmetic, because, it seemed, so many African women had unusually large clitoral or labial bulges. One scholar who traveled widely in Africa maintained that the sultry climate caused deformities of the female organs that rendered circumcision medically necessary. Indeed, the notion of a medical rationale for female circumcision dates back at least to the sixteenth century, when Catholic missionaries in Ethiopia sought to ban the practice among their converts as a throwback to paganism. The result, they soon learned to their consternation, was that uncircumcised Christian women were considered unmarriageable. This presented a serious obstacle to their proselytizing. But the problem was solved after a surgeon, sent from Rome as a consultant, concluded that the peculiarly large clitoris and labia of Ethiopian women were aberrant, provoking a natural aversion in men, and thus appropriate objects of surgical revision.[22]

Although the tradition underlying the practice was firmly upheld by men, the cutting itself was the work of women, usually older women. Exceptions to this rule certainly exist, but as Mohammed's dialogue with the exciser of slaves suggests, each sex circumcised its own. Sometimes, as with the Conibo tribes of Peru, the female circumciser worked alone: "an old woman, in the presence of the roaring tribe, performs it with a bamboo knife while the girl lies stretched out on three posts." Among the Elkoyni of equatorial Africa, the girl to be cut is bathed in the river by one woman, then publicly circumcised by an old woman. Afterward, she is confined to her hut, guarded by a company of village women.

The personal narratives of women who have been cut describe their abject powerlessness: being held down by women, one sitting on the chest, others gripping the arms and spreading the legs as the exciser commences her grim business. In effect, the picture is a group rape scene, with the girl violated and mutilated by those closest to her. In this nightmare tableau, the figure of the circumciser deserves comment. In Kassindja's case she was Rakia Idrissou, an elderly witch figure, red fingernails on gnarled fingers, whose office had been passed down from mother to daughter for generations. So, much as ritual cutting conformed to male dominance and tradition of the patriarchs, it also reinforced an important traditional role within the social structure of the tribe having to do with the dominance of one class of women over another. The older women, robbed of their own sexual sensitivity years earlier (and perhaps knowing that men preferred uncircumcised women as sexual partners) ensured that their daughters would not outstrip them. Thus they perpetuate a self-reinforcing cycle of suffering and loss.

A formidable obstacle for those who would ban female circumcision is that its victims usually accept it as necessary and desirable. In many communities, the clitoris is despised as thoroughly as American physicians spurn the male foreskin. Some myths teach that a man whose penis touches the clitoris may become ill or impotent. Others represent it as a source of potential danger to children: a baby whose head comes in contact with the clitoris may be born with excess cranial fluid; a mother whose baby touches the organ may find that her breast milk becomes poisonous. Like the foreskin, the clitoris and the labia are often seen as harbors of infection, including cancerous agents and sexually transmitted diseases.

In 1998, an anticircumcision activist posted a photograph of a young African girl on a web site. It carried the caption: "Should she be circumcised?"

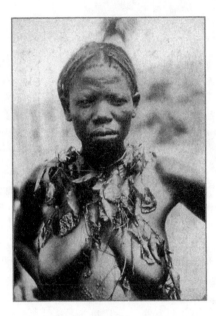

Village circum-
ciser, Zaire,
early 1930s.
From A. M.
Vergiat, *Les
Rites Secrets des
primitifs de
l'Oubangui*
(1936).

Plainly the answer was supposed to be no. But one response to the picture came from an African woman who had been circumcised as a girl and professed to be quite happy. "Circumcision has been popular among African women for many thousands of years," she wrote. "Western pressure groups attempt to blackmail African nations into banning the custom, but whenever moves are made to do this, the streets are filled with happy circumcised women demonstrating their desire to protect their daughters' right to enjoy the same benefits." She then proceeded to list more than a dozen "things that a girl gains when she is circumcised." These included:

- It is a rite of passage and proof of adulthood. One day she is a girl; the next a woman.
- It raises her status in her community, both because of the added purity that circumcision brings and the bravery that initiates are called upon to show.
- It confers maturity and inculcates positive character traits, including the ability to endure pain and a submissive nature.
- The circumcision ritual is an enjoyable one, in which the girl is the centre of attention and receives presents and moral instruction from her elders.
- It creates a bond between the generations, as all women in that society must undergo it and thus have shared an important experience.
- The girl will never have her conscience troubled by lustful thoughts or sensations or temptations such as masturbation.

She went on to say that by eliminating a woman's physical sex drive, circumcision made marriages more secure (the wife being drawn to her husband by love rather than lust), and thus provided greater stability for families. Perhaps Americans, with their high rates of crime and teenage pregnancy, had things backward. "Females are told that this little nub of skin, a vestigial penis, should have awesome phallic power," she concluded. "For most of them it just doesn't, which creates dissatisfaction."[23]

In a similar vein, a web site maintained by the Muslim Students' Association at the University of Houston in 1999 held that female circumcision, performed in accordance with Muslim law, continued to be desirable. "Some doctors and others try to belittle female circumcision and claim that it is harmful, an evil custom and is detrimental to health," the writers acknowledge. But when done properly, by specialists who do not cut "too severely," it actually produces substantial "health and psychological benefits." Women in warm climates, for instance, "may require circumcision since the hood of the clitoris may grow so large as to prevent sexual intercourse, or it may increase her desire when her clothes rub against it." Supposed medical benefits include fewer infections "resulting from microbes gathering under the hood of the clitoris," and a reduction in "attacks of herpes and genital ulcers."

Against charges of racism and cultural imperialism—that the animus against female circumcision springs from Westerners' desire to impose their values on the developing world—opponents of genital mutilation, male and female, have joined forces by sponsoring joint conferences, sharing mailing lists, and proclaiming a common rhetoric. Anyone familiar with the male anticircumcision movement will hear clear echoes in the language of Catherine Hogan, founder of the Washington Metropolitan Alliance Against Ritualistic FGM. "This is a clear case of child abuse," she maintained. "It's a form of reverse racism not to protect these girls from barbarous practices that rob them for a lifetime of their God-given right to an intact body."[24]

Such arguments proved persuasive in Europe and the United States. The United Kingdom and several other countries outlawed female genital mutilation, and in 1996 Congress passed legislation that established criminal penalties for cutting girls under eighteen years old. The same law provided funding for educational programs in African immigrant communities where female circumcision was practiced. During the mid-1990s, the medical groups whose members dealt with women's and children's health voiced uniform opposition. The American Medical Association, the American College of Obstetricians and Gynecologists, and the American Academy of Pediatrics each denounced "all medically unnecessary procedures to alter female genitalia." In

1998, AAP, whose statements about male circumcision had been models of ambiguity (leaving it to parents to decide whether their cultural preferences included removing their sons' foreskins), assailed female circumcision as child abuse and issued the following recommendations.

The American Academy of Pediatrics:

1. Opposes all forms of female genital mutilation (FGM).
2. Recommends that its members actively seek to dissuade families from carrying out FGM.
3. Recommends that its members provide patients and their parents with compassionate education about the physical harms and psychological risks of FGM.
4. Recommends that its members decline to perform any medically unnecessary procedure that alters the genitalia of female infants, girls, and adolescents.

Contrary to the way the academy approached male circumcision—appointing task forces made up of medical and surgical specialists—the policy on females was formulated by its Bioethics Committee, a group that had never been charged to review male circumcision.[25]

For decades, in the developing world most efforts to convert communities away from the practice have met with failure. Like male circumcision, the cutting of girls is an expression of certain deeply held beliefs about the body, human sexuality, and individual and social identity. Proponents of female circumcision like to point out that American parents circumcise their newborns so the sons will look like their fathers and other boys in the community. What, they ask, gives Americans the right to apply a different standard to African women?[26]

So far the most successful approach in persuading tribal communities to stop cutting girls has been a thoughtful educational program in Senegal. Rather than advancing the traditional moral arguments—that cutting is wrong because it hurts women, that it deprives women of sexual pleasure, and so forth—the international teams at work in Senegal have taken a different path. Village by village, a private Senegalese women's organization known as Tofhan puts on a series of two-month workshops focused principally on literacy, on broadening women's perspective to take in more of the modern world, and on health. "It started with basic reading and writing," said Rana Badri, who coordinated international opposition. "They didn't ask the community to stop the practice. This came as a result of the women's awareness of their rights." The program began with basic topics such as hygiene and childbirth. Slowly, as village women and instructors developed a common trust and frame of reference, talk about health blended into a discussion of human rights. The subject of female circumcision was not broached for a full year; and when it finally came up, it was entirely within the context of the procedure's health risks. Even though a number of Senegalese villages rejected the program as an intrusion into the most cherished rituals of their culture, in January 1999 the Parliament of Senegal, led by the country's president, Abdou Dious, voted to ban genital cutting of girls. This brought to more than a dozen the number of sub-Saharan African nations—including Burkina Faso, the Central African Republic, Djibouti, Ghana, Guinea, and Togo—that impose penalties for genital mutilation of girls.[27]

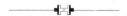

If female circumcision is mainly represented as a problem confined to developing nations, occasionally crossing onto American or European shores through immigration, a closer look at the record of Western medicine clouds the picture.

Before the turn of the century, Anglo-American physicians developed a variety of surgeries on female genitalia based on the same theory of reflex neurosis that justified circumcision in males. Some male surgeons simply had an "itch to cut," said the pioneering feminist physician Elizabeth Blackwell. The reasons for resecting a female organ that many physicians considered useless matched the rationale for removing the male foreskin: to prevent masturbation, sexually transmitted diseases, and cancer. During the Victorian period, a London surgeon named Isaac Baker Brown made a name for himself by excising the clitorises of women whose husbands thought them oversexed. And though he was drummed out of the Obstetrical Society of London for being too aggressive with the scalpel, Brown's practice and others like it thrived in United States. "Many women need circumcision," S. I. Kistler baldly told readers of the *Journal of the American Medical Association* in 1910.[28]

Through the 1950s, while aggressive surgeries like Baker's and Battey's "normal ovariotomy" fell by the wayside, surgeons continued to regard the clitoris with suspicion. The value of clitoral surgery "in improving function has been accepted by various cultures for 3,500 years," wrote surgeon W. G. Rathmann in a 1959 paper laying out what he regarded as the indications to operate. Borrowing terminology that had been used for nearly a century to describe problems of the male prepuce, Rathmann declared, "The two common problems that make the highly sensitive area of the clitoris unable to be stimulated are phimosis and redundancy." Others held more extreme views. "A clitoris is not necessary for normal sexual function," insisted a team of surgeons at a leading New York medical center in 1966 in their introduction to a punctilious guide to resecting it down to the root.[29]

Strangely enough, in the 1960s and 1970s surgery on the clitoris underwent a revival, though for precisely the opposite reasons it had formerly been applied. In 1973, calling attention to a growing trend, the mass circulation magazine *Playgirl* published an enthusiastic story headlined, "Circumcision for Women—The Kindest Cut of All." The story blazoned a practice endorsed by a number of physicians and enthusiastically touted by patients: the surgical peeling of part or the entire "foreskin" of the clitoris (the layers of tissue that hood the organ). Removing this excess skin, they claimed, made the clitoris more accessible to stimulation and thus heightened sexual response in women. Most physicians remained skeptical, however, and over the next several years opinion militated against the surgery. "Surgical procedures to enhance orgasmic response in the female are not effective," wrote a physician who had made a study of the published research, "and will invariably precipitate problems that are iatrogenic." Probably the most telling verdict was the decision of the commercial insurance industry to exclude female circumcision from coverage on the basis, according to a 1977 press release from the National Blue Shield Association, that the procedure was "obsolete or ineffective."[30]

Rates for many if not most surgical procedures done on women's reproductive organs are higher in the United States than in other industrialized countries. By the age of sixty, for example, one in three American women will have undergone hysterectomy to remove her uterus. In France, by contrast, the comparable figure is only one in eighteen. In some respects the debate over hysterectomy, and the value of the uterus as women age, resembles the circumcision controversy. Some physicians view the uterus as an incubator whose useful function ends when a woman delivers her last child. To this way of thinking, after childbearing the organ then becomes superfluous, and a prime target for disease. Alternatively, many researchers insist that the uterus continues to function into old age as a basic component of the body's endocrine system. They point out that it manufactures beta-endorphins, hormones regulating pain, along with prostacyclin, which keeps dangerous blood clots from forming inside veins. Critics of unnecessary hysterectomies list a series of harmful consequences. "The most frequent problems that women report are a loss of energy and stamina, loss of physical and sexual sensations," according to one activist. Even so, many doctors and women view hysterectomy as a quick, convenient, safe way to eliminate the pain and bleeding associated with fibroids (benign uterine growths) and endometriosis (protrusion of the uterus).[31]

During the 1980s and 1990s, the debate about the appropriate use of the scalpel on female genitalia took an unexpected turn. One by-product of media attention on female circumcision in Africa, along with a broader cultural trend that encouraged victims of all sorts of abuse to call attention to themselves, was the public appearance of a group of American women who claimed to have been subjected to mutilating genital surgery, albeit for medical reasons. "Africans have their cultural reasons for trimming girls' clitorises, and we have our cultural reasons for trimming girls' clitorises," declared Cheryl Chase, founder of the Intersex Society of North America. "It's a lot easier to see what's irrational in another culture than it is to see it in our own."[32]

The irrationality that Chase denounced has to do with the practice among pediatric surgeons of "correcting" ambiguous genitalia, often by cutting off part or all of a girl's clitoris if it is considered abnormally large or aesthetically repugnant. In some cases, congenital defects make it is impossible to classify a baby as female or male. Based on the diagnosis of ambiguous genitalia, or "intersexuality," doctors perform surgeries on some 2,000 children each year. Nine out of ten of these are classified as female, though this sex assignment may reflect little more than the surgeon's choice. Using the traditional techniques of plastic surgery, they endeavor to make the child look normal. This is where the trouble lies, with some activists accusing surgeons of operating far too aggressively with little sense of the lasting damage such procedures may do to women's lives. Depending on the extent of the surgery, women may be left with scars, numbness, and loss of sensation in their sexual organs, as well as with an abiding shame and embarrassment.

In the emotionally charged atmosphere of the female circumcision controversy, Chase dramatized intersexuality, displaying a knack for attracting media attention. (Her group's Internet web site promoted, among other things, a thirty-minute videotape entitled *Hermaphrodites Speak!*) Television and radio talk shows devoted hours of coverage to the subject. *Rolling Stone* published a long article chronicling "The True Story of John/Joan," a male baby who was badly maimed in a botched circumcision and as a result was "reassigned" to female sex, meaning that physicians performed plastic operations to fashion female genitalia, followed by hormone treatments to turn John into a girl. The article bitterly mocked the claim that physicians could manufacture gender, one of the central tenets of radical surgery for intersexuality.[33]

The medical debate over intersexuality is a microcosm of the debate over male circumcision. In 1997, a reporter for the *New York Times* interviewed doctors who insisted that surgery for ambiguous genitalia was usually medically appropriate for the baby and vital for the parents, who were typically horrified by what they saw. "I don't think it's an option for nothing to be done," said Anthony Caldamone, a pediatric urologist in Providence, Rhode Island. "I don't think parents can be told, this is a normal girl, and then have to be faced with what looks like an enlarged clitoris, or a penis, every time they change the diaper. We try to normalize the genitals to the gender to reduce psychosocial and functional problems later in life." Yet the reporter had no trouble finding a specialist who took an opposing view. "By the Hippocratic oath, you should first do no harm," said Justine Schober, a specialist in Pennsylvania. "And we can't say this surgery does no harm." Mightn't it just be possible, she asked, that a large clitoris amplified sexual pleasure?[34]

The question is reasonable. Yet, as with so many surgeries, the long-term outcomes of surgery for intersexuality are simply unknown. At Johns Hopkins University, a team of scientists has conducted experiments using an electromyograph to find out whether women who have undergone clitoral reduction surgery retain the capacity to transmit electrical impulses through their nerves. In the several cases they examined, the clitoris registered some response to electrical stimulus. But doubts remained as to whether this meant a woman could achieve normal arousal and orgasm. By 1997, it appeared that a more critical approach was moving into the mainstream of medicine. Johns Hopkins psychiatrist and former urologist William Reiner, for example, acknowledged that early surgery might produce more harm than good, that clitoral surgery ran risks of damage to sexual experience, and that gender engineered by surgery could not be reliably predicted.[35]

Meanwhile, feeling themselves maltreated by a medical establishment unprepared to take them seriously, Cheryl Chase's Intersex Society, armed with wrenching personal accounts of women who had been maimed as children, took their case to the halls of Congress. They aimed to strengthen the federal prohibition on female genital mutilation and make it apply to women like themselves, which they believed could be accomplished by adding a single word to the law. Pointing to a provision that allows for genital surgery in cases where it is "necessary to the health of the person on whom it is performed," they sought the qualification "physical health." This modification, they were convinced, would prevent physicians from operating, as Chase put it, "to prevent psychological and mental trauma for the child."

It is unlikely that such a measure would have any effect on the practice of the aptly named Gary Alter, a urologist and plastic surgeon in Los Angeles who in 1998 advertised "Female Genital Cosmetic Surgery." Alter explained this as "surgical procedures designed to improve the appearance of female genitalia . . . the ultimate way for women to be gorgeous absolutely everywhere." Along with a growing number of plastic surgeons in California, Alter has identified asymmetrical or larger-than-normal labia as a problem in need of a surgical solution. A reporter who interviewed Alter and reviewed before and after photographs of his handiwork wrote, "What strikes me in the 'after' shots is the eerie similarity between the women. Pre-op, you could have picked their labia out of a lineup; now, their genitalia are carbon copies of each other."[36]

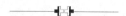

At the beginning of the twenty-first century, in a world that is preoccupied more than ever with health, and with extraordinary horizons visible in biotechnology, genomics, and genetic medicine, female circumcision is bound to seem atavistic. Stripped of medical or scientific support, it is now viewed as the province of the unenlightened, an outrageous throwback to primitive ideas about women, disregarding women's suffering and their right to control their bodies. Our revulsion toward cutting the genitals of girls should give us pause, however, for the themes the Western world abhors—removing part of the genitals to reduce sexual pleasure, carving children's bodies to conform to certain social ideals, visiting pain on helpless children—are all fully present in the history of male circumcision.

Many people find the analogy disconcerting. Most Americans, even those who consider male circumcision unnecessary, cannot help but think of the circumcised penis as normal and the foreskin as a piece of excess skin. Much as we believe ourselves to be enlightened citizens of the age of science, not superstition, the continuing circumcision of newborn American boys betrays lingering illusions about health and reveals the power of culture in shaping medical practice. Egyptians and ancient Israelites and Australian bushmen wove stories about gods, the redemptive power of spilt blood, totems, and so on, thereby enshrining the cutting of the penis as a terrible and momentous ritual connected to man's fate within the cosmos. The modern age in turn reinvented the ritual, substituting for older religious ideas its own set of moral mythologies in the guise of medicine. In place of the old taboos, circumcision was justified as protection against the dread diseases of modern civilization: cancer, syphilis, and AIDS. Science has slowly discredited theories that give circumcision any meaningful role as a public health measure; yet even today many American doctors continue to use science to promote health fantasies about the procedure.

Surgery requires a confidence that borders on faith. In order to operate, surgeons convince themselves that the patient will be better off for their efforts. (This applies to religious operators as much as doctors.) The history of surgery, however, is rife with examples of false confidence. In 1936, the Portuguese neurologist Egas Moniz pioneered an operation to sever the brain's frontal lobes from its centers of emotion. Thirteen years later, the frontal lobotomy was so well accepted that Moniz shared the Nobel Prize in medicine for inventing it. The more the operation was used, however, the clearer it became that its long-term mental results were devastating. By the late 1950s, surgeons abandoned lobotomy. Over the next decade or so, tonsillectomy fell out of vogue. Hysterectomy, caesarean sections, prostate gland removal, all fads in America at the end of the twentieth century, are likely to decline in favor in the decades to come. It is likely that, deprived of its scientific legitimacy and at the same time steadily diminished as a mark of social distinction, routine medical circumcision will go the way of routine bloodletting.

Ultimately, the enigma of circumcision is less how it came to be in the first place than how, having been invented, it has survived so long. In Judaism and Islam, the answer is that circumcision is the symbol of belonging to God's chosen people. Although the trappings of the rituals and many of the lesser meanings of circumcision vary from group to group, it reflects a powerful historical continuity back to a common patriarch, Abraham; its enduring power exemplifies faith and religious community.

From a different perspective, the mark of the covenant also helps illuminate the American transformation of circumcision from a religious ritual to an enduring secular custom. Since the earliest period of their history, Americans have identified with the Old Testament along with the New. They have shared an extraordinary sense of destiny. Approaching the New World, John Winthrop, in his unforgettable sermon *A Modell of Christian Charity* (1630), told his fellow Puritans, "We must consider that we shall be as a city upon a hill. The eyes of all people are upon us." Over the next three centuries, through the forming of a nation and the trial by fire of the Civil War, American ideology embraced the idea that, in the divine scheme of history, America had succeeded Israel.

The United States became the new Promised Land. The religious core of American culture remained Protestant, but from the era of the founding fathers it also developed an important secular dimension: a common national creed and intellectual idiom that has been called America's "civil religion." Evidence of this generic religiosity is everywhere, from presidential discourse to the inscription In God We Trust on the copper penny. Ironically, circumcision, converted more than a century ago from a religious tenet to medical wisdom, has marked generations of males born in the United States not as the children of Israel but, in Lincoln's astute phrase, God's "almost chosen people."

APPENDIX:

Evaluative Research and the

Nature of Medical Evidence

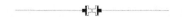

Because the medical circumcision debate has grown so heated, it is useful to review what physicians agree on. First, everyone concedes that the foreskin cannot be the cause of diseases that occur in both uncircumcised and circumcised males. Most men, whatever their state, remain free from diseases associated with the foreskin.

If not a direct antecedent of disease, though, the foreskin could be a risk factor, something that increases the odds of a man's developing one or more disorders. Indeed, most of the medical literature revolves around risk factors, yet the problem is how to calculate their relative influence. A high level of HDL cholesterol is commonly understood to be a pressing risk factor for coronary artery disease; the higher the level, the greater the hazard. Moderate consumption of alcohol, in contrast, may or may not be a risk factor. Older studies indicated a weak link between drinking and heart disease, but more recent studies have shown that drinking moderate amounts of alcohol, particularly red wine, confers protective benefits (though the physiochemistry of the protective effect remains cryptic). While the latter studies are better designed, both sets suffer from a common problem: namely, the weaker the risk factor, the weaker the evidence, thus the harder to demonstrate any effect conclusively.

What intellectual tools are available to ascertain how any surgery affects patients? The oldest and still the most widely applied is expert opinion, the judgment of physicians based on experience with patients. Of more recent vintage is the randomized controlled trial, which has become the standard for testing the safety and efficacy of new medicines at the U.S. Food and Drug Administration (FDA). The evidence marshaled by most papers published in peer-reviewed journals (an eclectic category characterized by enormous variations in scientific standards) falls somewhere in between these two approaches. Most of the time we are confronted by case reports (often of just one case), clinical series, nonrandomized controlled trials, case-control studies, and meta-analyses (an increasingly popular avenue of research that combines and abstracts data from multiple studies).

It is essential to remember that for any surgical procedure applied to large populations there is variation, often wide variation, with respect to its benefits and harms.

Patients differ, surgeons vary, circumstances and environments are never exactly the same. All this variation means that, as we generalize from individuals to populations, the best we can do is to estimate the approximate magnitude of a procedure's effects, good and bad. Precisely because estimates can be more or less accurate, a requisite component of any proper analysis is to pinpoint the estimates' range of uncertainty.

In technical terms, the methods for appraising clinical studies or medical journal articles hinge on a handful of basic statistical concepts and techniques: sample size, confidence intervals, probability distributions, odds ratios, and so forth. They also involve detecting bias. Fundamentally, there are two kinds of bias—to internal and to external validity—that influence clinical evaluative research. Internal validity has to do with how accurately a study estimates outcomes within the strict context of the research design itself. Biases to internal validity mean that, if a study is designed to demonstrate how circumcision relates to a specific indication—for example, urinary tract infection (UTI) among white males between the ages of four weeks and twelve months—how accurately do the findings characterize that specific group and setting? In contrast, external validity biases determine how well the findings of one study translate to other settings and other populations.[1] Depending on its gravity, bias has the potential to warp research that on its surface appears extremely convincing.

The most common bias to internal validity in circumcision research is a product of patient selection. In hundreds of studies, groups of circumcised and uncircumcised males have been compared with respect to some medical diagnosis—sexually transmitted disease infection, for example—and the two groups are evaluated against each other as if they were the same in all respects, except the presence or absence of a prepuce. It was on this basis that many nineteenth-century physicians concluded that because Jews suffered lower rates of syphilis than other immigrant groups, circumcision offered protection against venereal disease. Such logic is deceptive. Circumcision has never been applied randomly. As one team of social scientists recently put it: "There are strongly associated social and behavioral co-variants with circumcision status that include social background characteristics, such as age, education, race/ethnicity, and sexual practices and preferences. In short, circumcision is a marker for a complex array of social and behavioral characteristics."[2]

There are always underlying social and cultural differences between circumcised and uncircumcised populations. These are hard to describe, and even harder to estimate in terms of their health implications. Yet these deep-seated differences may be far more relevant to a certain diagnosis than circumcision.

Other examples of biases to internal validity include inaccuracies in determining who was circumcised or not for study purposes, and errors in measuring outcomes. In retrospective studies, for instance, many researchers have complained that circumcision is not always indicated in a patient's medical chart. The omission rate has been estimated as high as 15 percent. Moreover, in studies based on self-reported rates of circumcision, many men are either ignorant of or mistaken about their own circumcision status. Particularly with older men, errors creep in owing to cloudy memories and missing records. Other research adds to the confusion by claiming that *when* a male was circumcised—in infancy, youth, or adulthood—matters. Outcomes present an especially knotty problem. The medical benefits claimed for circumcision are mainly preventive. So the presumptive surgical outcome is not developing a certain disease. The trouble is, with the exception of diseases of the foreskin itself, circumcised and uncircumcised males suffer the same diseases, albeit at different rates.

Two types of biases to external validity permeate circumcision studies. First is what epidemiologists call *population bias*. This occurs when there are significant differences between the groups actually studied and the populations to whom researchers want to apply their conclusions. How confident, for instance, can one be in projecting findings about HIV infection from a study of long-distance truck drivers in Kenya to the male population of the United States or Germany? A lesser though hardly insignificant problem is termed *intensity bias*. This means that a procedure that is nominally the same may, owing to variations in technique, medical technology, and the skill of the surgeons who perform it, differ in important ways from patient to patient or group to group. Circumcision, in other words, is not always the same operation. Technical discrepancies in how it is performed and by whom (pediatrician, obstetrician, *mohel* et al.) may influence outcomes as well.

We are unlikely to see a large randomized prospective study. It is hard to imagine parents placing their babies in a research pool for random assignment to a circumcision or noncircumcision group. So we are stuck with cohort studies, case-control studies, and anecdotes.

Not that these are useless, but to deal with their relative biases and uncertainties it helps to apply consistent, reasonable standards of evidence. These include:

- What is the study's evidence? How do we estimate its bias? What must be done to adjust for this bias?
- If the bias is acceptable, does the study demonstrate that circumcision has any effect at all, no matter how minor, on the disease in question?
- If the results are ambiguous, how do we weigh the value of rejecting a procedure that may be beneficial against accepting one that may be worthless?

A typical cohort study begins with matched groups of healthy circumcised and uncircumcised men. Each group is followed for the period of the study, with researchers examining the men for symptoms of disease. The observation that the uncircumcised group had a higher incidence of STDs would be consistent with the hypothesis that circumcision reduces the risk of STD infection. The mirror image of this approach is the case-control method in which, to use a similar example, researchers assemble a group of healthy patients, designated as a control group, and another group diagnosed with STDs. They proceed to check the incidence of circumcision in each group. Again, if the infected group had a higher incidence of circumcision than the control group, it would support the hypothesis that the foreskin is a risk factor in STD infection. In either method, the difference in STD infection would be expressed as the *odds ratio* of an uncircumcised man's being infected versus his circumcised counterpart. An odds ratio of 1.0 would mean that the two groups were infected at the same rate. An odds ratio of 2.0, that uncircumcised men were twice as likely to be infected, or 0.5, half as likely. If the populations were perfectly matched, with circumcision being the only salient difference, the greater the odds ratio, the greater the chance that circumcision (or uncircumcision) would be a risk factor.

The conceptual and emotional problems of sorting out medical risks and benefits are apparent in two recent controversies, both related to women's breasts. The first of these was the infamous silicone gel implant case. Though lacking any scientific evidence that silicone implants caused disease, the FDA chose to pull them off the market. This action opened the way for a barrage of product liability lawsuits. Tens of thousands of women blamed their implants for a bewildering array of maladies. Juries tended to side with plaintiffs. Yet when careful epidemiological studies were published, there was little solid evidence that silicone posed the health dangers women and their lawyers claimed.[3]

A different problem of assessing risk surfaced in the dispute over whether women in their forties should get routine mammograms to screen for cancer. While breast cancer is a leading cause of death in this age group, an expert panel assembled by the National Institutes of Health (NIH) decided against regular screening. The reasoning went like this: at most, the procedure might save the life of 1 out of every 1,000 women examined. But there would be a very high rate of false-positive mammograms. Many women in their forties have noncancerous masses in their breasts. Judging by mammogram images alone, in many cases doctors simply could not tell whether a small lump was benign or malignant. So, in order to be sure (and protect themselves from malpractice liability), they would have to subject women to biopsies. In addition to many unnecessary surgeries, routine mammograms would probably trigger cancer in some women—perhaps 3 in 10,000—by exposing them to X rays. Taken together, the panel concluded, the actual benefits of regular mammography for women under fifty were miniscule, so tiny, as one critic put it, that "the risks of driving the car to get them might well outweigh the benefits of the test."[4]

This scientific conclusion cut little ice with many women's groups and medical professionals who had come to view mammography as a powerful weapon in the battle against breast cancer. Scorning the notion that "only" 1 woman in 1,000 would be saved ("What if that one woman was you or your wife," went a common refrain), advocates pressured the NIH to appoint a second panel that, unsurprisingly, reversed the original decision. Lost in the popular media coverage that did so much to inflame the issue was the fact that breast cancer attacks fewer than 2 percent of women between forty and forty-nine, and that detecting a tumor early improves but by no means assures a woman's hope of cure.

With mammography, as with much of medicine, multiple studies fail to provide an absolute answer. In truth, only a small minority of women will ever be physically affected by mammography. Alternatively, many will be affected psychologically, whether suffering through the worries of a false positive or catching a treatable tumor in time to save life or breast.

NOTES

⁜

PREFACE

1. D. M. Eddy, television interview, BBC Science Features, January 1992, quoted in M. Konner, *Medicine at the Crossroads: The Crisis in Health Care* (1993), 137.

CHAPTER ONE

1. J. Pritchard, ed., *Ancient Near Eastern Texts Relating to the Old Testament* (1950), 326.

2. A. Badawy, *The Tomb of Nyhetep-Ptah at Giza and the Tomb of Ankhmahor at Saqqara* (1978), 19; A. Cockburn and E. Cockburn, eds., *Mummies, Disease, and Ancient Cultures*, vol. 1 (1980), 18, 42; H. Sigerist, *A History of Medicine*, vol. 1. *Primitive and Archaic Medicine* (1950), 345.

3. P. Ghalioungui, *Magic and Medical Science in Ancient Egypt* (1963), 95, 150; W. Burkert, *Creation of the Sacred: Tracks of Biology in Early Religions* (1996).

4. One scholar has even suggested that the famous images in the Tomb of Ankhmahor represent medical treatment, with physicians operating on patients for phimosis. See C. de Wit, "Le circoncision chez les anciens Égyptiens," *Zeitschrift für Ägyptische Sprache 99* (1972): 41–48.

5. G. Majno, *The Healing Hand: Man and Wound in the Ancient World* (1975), 97.

6. J. Harris and K. Weeks, *X-raying the Pharaohs* (1973), 126–30; R. Porter, *The Greatest Benefit to Mankind: A Medical History of Humanity* (1998), 49. Assigning circumcision to a particular group of priests or physicians would have been consistent with Egypt's penchant for specialization. Within the Egyptian medical world in the fifth century B.C., the Greek historian Herodotus commented to the unusual division of labor, with physicians devoting themselves to particular organs and disorders.

7. J. Estes, *The Medical Skills of Ancient Egypt* (1989), 155–57.

8. Freud's interpretation is set forth in *Moses and Monotheism* (1939).

9. P. Machinist, "The Meaning of Moses," *Harvard Divinity Bulletin 27* (1998): 15.

10. H. Eilberg-Schwartz, *The Savage in Judaism: An Anthropology of Israelite Religion and Ancient Judaism* (1990), 142–43.

11. K. Kohler, "Circumcision," *Jewish Encyclopedia*, vol. 4 (1903): 92–96; N. J. McEleney, "Conversion, Circumcision and the Law," *New Testament Studies* (1974): 319–41; G. Lerner, *The Creation of Patriarchy* (1986), 192.

12. Eilberg-Schwartz, *Savage in Judaism*, 148.

13. During the flight from Egypt, for instance, God tells Moses to prepare a Passover offering, charging him, "If a stranger who dwells with you would offer the Passover to the Lord, all his males must be circumcised. But no uncircumcised person may eat of it" (Exodus 12:48).

14. In some versions, the word *uncircumcised* is mistranslated as "forbidden."

15. Eilberg-Schwartz, *Savage in Judaism*, 152.

16. The emphasis on blood captured the attention of early anthropologists. See R. Andree, "Beschneidung," *Ethnographishe Parallelen* (1899), 166–212; and for the claim that circumcision is a "blood covenant" see A. J. Reinach, "La lutte de Jacob et de Moïse avec Jahvé et l'origine de la circoncision," *Revue des Études ethnologiques et sociologiques* (1908): 360–62.

17. Philo, *The Works of Philo*, vol. 3, trans. C. Yonge (1993), 48.

18. Philo, *Questions and Answers on Genesis*, ed. R. Marcus (1971), 244, 251; Philo, *The Special Laws*, vol. 1, trans. F. H. Colson (1937), 8–9.

19. For an excellent overview see P. Schäfer, *Judeophobia: Attitudes Toward the Jews in the Ancient World* (1998).

20. Quoted in J. Cooper, *The Child in Jewish History* (1996), 51.

21. L. Ginzberg, *Legends of the Jews*, vol. 6 (1909–1938), 24n141.

22. Quoted in M. L. Barth, "Berit Milah in Midrash and Agada," in L. M. Barth, ed., *Berit Milah in the Reform Context* (1990), 104–12.

23. A. Edwardes, *Erotica Judaica* (1967), 109–10.

24. S. Zeitlin, *The Rise and Fall of the Judean State,* vol. 2 (1967), 202.

25. Described in Bergson, *Die Beschneidung* (1844), 13. The most detailed account of the technique involved is in J. P. Rubin, "Celsus' Decircumcision Operation," *Urology 16* (1980): 124.

26. The passage is from the "Mishnah and Herbert Danby" (451:13), quoted in *Writings from Rabbi Schnur: Ritual Circumcision.* The origins of *periah* have long been a matter of disagreement. Some orthodox rabbis, seeking precedents in the era of the patriarchs, have suggested that it dates back to Joshua, relying on a rather strained interpretation of God's commandment "circumcise a second time" (Joshua 5:2).

27. *Pirkei de Rabbi Eliezer*, ch. 29, cited in L. A. Hoffman, *Covenant of Blood: Circumcision and Gender in Rabbinic Judaism* (1996), 102. This discussion of the centrality of blood to circumcision ritual and symbolism in Rabbinic Judaism is drawn from Hoffman's excellent study.

28. *Seder Rav Amram Gaon*, ed. E. D. Goldschmidt (1971), 180; Isefer Ha'Eshkol, *Hilchot milah*, Auerbach ed. (1868), 131.

29. The literature on gender bias in Judaism is extensive. On the narrower issue of blood duality and how circumcision worked to circumscribe women's role in Jewish religious life, see L. J. Archer, "Bound by Blood: Circumcision and Menstrual Taboo in Post-Exilic Judaism," in Y. Y. Haddad and E. Findly, eds., *After Eve* (1985), 8–9; R. Wasserfall, "Menstruation and Identity: The Meaning of *Niddah* for Moroccan Women Immigrants in Israel," in H. Eilberg-Schwartz, ed., *People of the Body: Jews and Judaism from an Embodied Perspective* (1992).

30. A. Cohen, *Everyman's Talmud* (1975), 381; Avoth 3:15.

31. *The Wisdom of the Zohar: An Anthology of Texts*, vol. 3, ed. I. Tishby, trans. D. Goldstein

(1989), 1176, 1181. There is an interesting parallel between Rabbi Simeon's notion that the blood spilled in circumcision precipitates God's forgiveness and the Christian idea that the blood of Christ, shed at his crucifixion, atoned for the sins of humankind.

32. M. Maimonides, *Guide to the Perplexed*, vol. 3, trans. S. Pines, 8.

33. Ibid., 49.

34. Maimonides, *Guide to the Perplexed*, 3:8.

35. Midrash Tadshe 8, 152.

36. Quoted in M. Saperstein, *Decoding the Rabbis* (1980), 98. See also D. Biale, *Eros and the Jews: From Biblical Israel to Contemporary America* (1997), 94–95.

37. *Shivhei ha-Ran*, sec. 16, 18, quoted in Biale, *Eros and the Jews*, 134.

38. R. Rosenthal, "The Care of the Sick in the Bible and the Talmud," in S. R. Kagan, ed., *Victor Robinson Memorial Volume* (1948), 353–58.

39. Quoted in F. Rosner, *Medicine in the Bible and in the Talmud: Selections from Classical Jewish Sources* (1977), 46–47.

40. *Preuss' Biblical and Talmudic Medicine*, trans. F. Rosner (1978), 240–48; F. Rosner, *Medicine in the Mishneh Torah of Maimonides* (1984), 263–71; S. R. Kagan, *Jewish Medicine* (1952), 562; F. Rosner, "Hemophilia in the Talmud and Rabbinic Writings," *Annals of Internal Medicine 70* (1969), 833–37.

41. "Essay," *Sichos in English* (1998), 3. Rabbi Chassidus maintained that the foreskin acted as a barrier to divine illumination, which he termed "arousal from Above." *Berit milah*, he said, "draws down a level of the soul that transcends intellect." Chassidus, "Tazria: Circumcision—Always a Timely Act," *Likkutei Sichos 3* (n.d.): 979.

42. D. J. Lasker, "Transubstantiation, Elijah, Plato, and the Jewish-Christian Debate," *Revue des Études Juives 143* (1984): 31–58. During the Renaissance, there was vigorous debate over the symbolic presence of Elijah at the circumcision ceremony and its meaning.

43. F. Bryk, *Circumcision in Man and Woman* (1934), 49. Bryk's account is drawn from H. Ploss, *Das Kind in Brauch und Sitte der Voelker* (1884).

44. Ibid., 49.

45. I. G. Marcus, *Rituals of Childhood: Jewish Acculturation in Medieval Europe* (1996), 105–7. The bar mitzvah rite, whereby a boy at the age of thirteen years and a day was acknowledged to enter maturity (and thus become eligible for certain religious duties, such as fasting), did not appear until the fifteenth century.

46. J. Buxtorf, *Synagoga Judaica/Das ist Jüden Schul* (1603), quoted in E. Horowitz, "The Eve of Circumcision: A Chapter in the History of Jewish Nightlife," *Journal of Social History 23* (1989): 47. Horowitz construes these ceremonies as examples of popular religion subsuming central rituals of Judaism, similar to the populism that transformed the principal symbols and rituals of Christianity during the same period.

47. Quoted in A. Berliner, *Geschichte der Juden in Rom* (1893), 11–12.

48. E. Horowitz, "The Even of Circumcision," *Journal of Social History 23* (1989): 60. Unfortunately Horowitz, except to note the ultimate triumph of the reformers, is at something of a loss to explain why the joyous (if occasionally intemperate) precircumcision ceremonies died out.

49. This incident occurred at a time when Christian public health authorities were trying to restrict *mohels*, who had been implicated in spreading disease, by outlawing genital surgery except when practiced by a licensed practitioner. See Hoffman, *Covenant of Blood*, 5–8.

50. Quoted in D. Philipson, *The Reform Movement in Judaism* (1907), 136.

51. Hoffman, *Covenant of Blood*, 9.

52. J. Helfand, "A German Mohel in Revolutionary France," *Revue des Études Juives 143* (1984): 365–71; R. S. Wolper, "Circumcision as Polemic in the Jew Bill of 1753: The Cutter Cut?" *Eighteenth-Century Life* 7 (1982): 28–36; D. M. G. Salomon, *Die Beschneidung: Historisch und Medizinisch Braunschweig* (1844), 48–49.

53. L. Lagnado, "Rabbis Mulling a Mystery of AIDS and Mohels," *Forward*, 18 August 1995.

CHAPTER 2

1. J. Marcus, "The Circumcision and the Uncircumcision in Rome," *New Testament Studies 35* (1989): 75. Marcus convincingly argues that many passages in the Bible customarily translated using the words *circumcision* or *uncircumcision* are in fact more specific, with *circumcision*, for example, really meaning "circumcised glans."

2. N. J. McEleney, "Conversion, Circumcision and the Law," *New Testament Studies 20* (1974): 339.

3. Abelard, *Dialogue of a Philosopher with a Jew and a Christian*, Pontifical Institute of Medieval Studies, *Sources in Translation*, vol. 20 (1979).

4. Abelard, *Sermon on Circumcision*, quoted in A. S. Abulafia, *Christians and Jews in the Twelfth-Century Renaissance* (1986), 125; J. L. Thompson, "'So Ridiculous a Sign': Men, Women, and the Lessons of Circumcision in Sixteenth-Century Exegesis," *Archiv für Reformationsgeschichte 86* (1996): 236–56. Thompson shows that early Protestant commentators shared with their Catholic forebears a desire to vaunt the superiority of the New Testament over the Old while at the same time maintaining historical continuity from Adam through Christ to the sixteenth-century church.

5. St. Thomas Aquinas, *Summa Theologica*, vol. 3: 70, 4.

6. A. Muller, *Die "hochheilige" Vorhaut Christi, im Kult und in der Theologie der Papstkirche* (1907), 51.

7. W. Cumming, ed. and trans., *The Revelations of Saint Birgitta* (1971).

8. P. Dinzelbacher and R. Vogeler, eds. and trans., *Leben un Offenbarungen der Wiener Begine Agnes Blannbekin* (1994). Eating the foreskin after circumcision, primarily as a token of fertility, is not uncommon in rituals from Africa to Australia.

9. F. Bryk, *Circumcision in Man and Woman* (1934), 25.

10. Quoted in J. Shapiro, *Shakespeare and the Jews* (1992), 4.

11. Quoted in J. Arnold, "The Jews in Medieval Society," Lecture given at the University of East Anglia, 17 May 1999.

12. J. Jacob, ed., *The Jews of Angevin England* (1893); J. R. Marcus, ed., *The Jew in the Medieval World* (1975).

13. S. Grayzel, *The Church and the Jews in the XIIIth Century*, vol. 2. *1254–1314*, ed. K. R. Stow (1989), 246.

14. C. Fabre-Vassas, *The Singular Beast: Jews, Christians, & the Pig* (1998), quoted in E. Horowitz, "Impurity and Danger," *The New Republic*, 8 June 1998, 42.

15. J. Shapiro, *Shakespeare and the Jews* (1992), 14.

16. Quoted in ibid., 17.

17. J. Bodenschatz, *Kirchliche Verfassung der huetigen Juden* (1749), 67.

18. R. Crashaw, "Our Lord in His Circumcision to His Father," in *The Verse in English of Richard Crashaw* (1949), 50.

19. *John Milton: Complete Poems and Major Prose*, ed. M. Y. Hughes (1957), 80–81.

20. M. an-Asimi, *The Medicine of the Prophet and Modern Science* (1977); M. ad-Duqr and M. al-Quwatli, "Circumcision and Medicine in Islam," *Civilization of Islam 14* (1983), 7.

21. Unlike his Jewish predecessors, however, al-Sukkari failed to ask why, if the foreskin were an imperfection, God had created it in the first place.

22. A. abu-Sahlieh, *To Mutilate in the Name of Jehovah or Allah: Legitimization of Male and Female Circumcision* (1994), 6.

23. W. R. Smith, *Lectures on the Religion of the Semites* (1927), 328.

24. T. V. N. Persaud and M. A. Ahmed, "Sunan Al-Fitra and Rules of Cleanliness in Islam," presented at the First International Conference for the Scientific Aspects of the Qur'an and Sunnah, Islamabad, Pakistan, 1987.

25. P. J. Imperato, *African Folk Medicine: Practices and Beliefs of the Bambara and Other Peoples* (1977), 188–89.

26. V. A. Naipaul, *Beyond Belief: Islamic Excursions Among the Converted Peoples* (1998). For a masterful portrait of the Islamizing process in one section of Indonesia, see C. Geertz, *Islam Observed* (1968).

27. R. Levy, *The Social Structure of Islam* (1957), 251–52.

28. E. Marx, "Circumcision Feasts Among the Negev Bedouins," *International Journal of Middle East Studies 4* (1973): 411–27. See also V. W. Turner, "Three Symbols of Passage in Ndembu Circumcision Ritual: An Interpretation," in M. Gluckman, ed., *Essays on the Ritual of Social Relations* (1962).

29. Marx, "Circumcision Feasts," 423–24.

30. Ibid., 425; Turner, "Three Symbols of Passage," 144.

31. Abu-Sahlieh, *To Mutilate in the Name of Jehovah or Allah*, 4–6.

32. A clear case study outlining the transformation of pre-Islamic rituals in western Nigeria is Mo. O. Adeleye, "Impacts of Islam on Some Social Features of Ijesa People of Nigeria," *Islamic Quarterly 31* (1993): 63–72. See also J. S. Trimingham, *The Influence of Islam upon Africa*, 2d ed. (1980), 70–71; I. A. Mansurnoor, *Islam in an Indonesian World: Ulama of Madura* (1990), 70–73.

33. M. R. Woodward, *Islam in Java: Normative Piety and Mysticism in the Sultanate of Yogyakarta* (1989), 160–63.

34. Abu-Sahlieh, *To Mutilate in the Name of Jehovah or Allah*, 8.

CHAPTER THREE

1. One of the earliest works that grapples with the problem of tribal circumcision in the context of biblical literalism is A. C. Borheck, *Is die Beschneidung ursprunglich hebraeisch? Und was veranlasste den Abraham zu ihrer Einfuhrung?* (1793).

2. For an excellent overview of Burton's life and work see M. S. Lovell, *A Rage to Live: A Biography of Richard and Isabel Burton* (1999); A. Lang, *Myth, Ritual, and Religion*, 2 vols. (1891). The first edition of James G. Frazer's influential book *The Golden Bough* was a two-

volume work published in London in 1890. Subsequently, beginning in 1906, *The Golden Bough* would swell to twelve volumes. Frazer's explanation of circumcision was published as "The Origin of Circumcision," *Independent Review* 4 (1904–5): 204–18.

3. Frazer, *The Golden Bough*.

4. M. Eliade, *Rites and Symbols of Initiation* (1958), 23.

5. A. van Gennep, *Les Rites de passage* (1908); English edition, *The Rites of Passage*, trans. M. Vizedom and G. Caffee, intro. S. T. Kimball (1960). In addition to coining the term *rite of passage*, van Gennep laid out what he called the rite's classic *schéma* or pattern: separation, transition, and incorporation.

6. van Gennep, *Rites of Passage* (1960), 71–72. While the general outline of van Gennep's interpretation fits Israel, he thoroughly rejected the notion that shedding of blood was integral to the ritual (p. 72*n*1).

7. J. La Fontaine, *Initiation* (1985), 113.

8. For an example of the adaptation of van Gennep's typology, see M. Gluckman, "The Roles of the Sexes in Wiko Circumcision Ceremonies," in M. Fortes, ed., *Social Structure: Studies Presented to A. R. Radcliffe-Brown* (1949); B. Malinowski, *Magic, Science and Religion and Other Essays* (1948), 21.

9. B. Spencer and F. J. Gillen, *The Arunta: A Study of a Stone Age People* (1927); H. Basedow, *The Australian Aboriginal* (1925).

10. The concept of "primitive culture," albeit widely used, is oversimplified and inadequate. For an illuminating discussion see C. Geertz, *After the Fact: Two Countries, Four Decades, One Anthropologist* (1955), 42–63.

11. M. F. Ashley-Montagu, *Coming into Being Among the Australian Aborigines: A Study of the Procreative Beliefs of the Native Tribes of Australia* (1937), 40–42.

12. Basedow, *Australian Aboriginal*, 243.

13. M. F. Ashley-Montagu, "Ritual Mutilation Among Primitive Peoples," *Ciba Symposia* (1946): 423–24.

14. M. F. Ashley-Montagu, "Mutilated Humanity," *Humanist* 55 (1995): 12–17.

15. The account that follows is based on M. Bloch, *From Blessing to Violence: History and Ideology in the Circumcision Ritual of the Merina of Madagascar* (1986), 48–83.

16. B. Bettelheim, *Sacred Wounds: Puberty Rites and the Envious Male* (1955), 160; E. Westermarck, *Ritual and Belief in Morocco*, vol. 2 (1926), 426–27.

17. G. de Buffon, *Voyage de Gemelli Careri*, vol. 2 (1719), 200; F. Bryk, *Circumcision in Man and Woman: Its History, Psychology and Ethnology*, trans. D. Berger (1934), 31; M. Leris and A. Schaeffner, "Les Rites de Circoncision Chez les Dogon de Sanga," *Journal de la Société des Africanistes* 6 (1936): 141–61.

18. For context see J. Hartke, "Castrating the Phallic Mother: The Influence of Freud's Repressed Developmental Experiences on the Conceptualization of the Castration Complex," *Psychoanalytic Review* 81 (1994): 641–57.

19. S. Freud, *Sexuality in the Etiology of the Neuroses* (1898), 278.

20. S. Freud, *Moses and Monotheism* (1939), 192; *New Introductory Lectures on Psychoanalysis* (1933), 120–21. From time to time, Freud voiced misgivings about this fantastic, undocumented primal event, yet in his final summation of psychoanalytic theory he wrote, "The possibility cannot be excluded that a phylogenetic memory may contribute to the extraordinarily terrifying effect of the threat [of castration]—a memory trace from the pre-

history of the human family, when the jealous father would actually rob his son of his genitals if the latter interfered with him in rivalry for a woman. The primeval custom of circumcision, another symbolic substitute for castration, is only intelligible if it is an expression of subjection to the father's will. (Compare the puberty rites of primitive peoples.)" See *An Outline of Psychoanalysis* (1949), 92–93.

21. T. Reik, *Ritual: Psycho-Analytic Studies* (1946); J. W. M. Whiting, R. Kluckholn, and A. Anthony, "The Function of Male Initiation Ceremonies at Puberty," in E. E. MacCoby et al., eds., *Readings in Social Psychology* (1958).

22. H. Nunberg, *Problems of Bisexuality as Reflected in Circumcision* (1949), 1.

23. F. Zimmerman, "Origin and Significance of the Jewish Rite of Circumcision," *Psychoanalytic Review 38* (1951): 112.

24. G. Cansever, "Psychological Effects of Circumcision," *British Journal of Medical Psychology 38* : 321–31.

25. Bettelheim, *Symbolic Wounds*, 26.

26. Since Bettelheim's suicide in 1990 at the age of eighty-six, his once-bright reputation has been eclipsed by evidence of mendacity and, more seriously, sadistic treatment of patients under his care. Psychologists remain divided over the value of his insights. For a balanced, if sympathetic, treatment of his life, see N. Sutton, *Bettelheim: A Life and a Legacy* (1995); Bettelheim, *Symbolic Wounds*, 116.

27. Bettelheim, *Symbolic Wounds*, 27–45, 261.

28. P. Erny, *Childhood and Cosmos: The Social Psychology of the Black African Child* (1974). The reconciliation in marriage of masculine-feminine duality in several of these myths recalls Plato's *Symposium*.

29. C. Geertz, *Works and Lives* (1988), 147.

CHAPTER FOUR

1. L. A. Sayre, "Partial Paralysis from Reflex Irritation, Caused by Congenital Phimosis and Adherent Prepuce," *Transactions of the American Medical Association 23* (1870): 205.

2. Ibid.,

3. Ibid., 205–6.

4. Ibid., 206.

5. Ibid., 206–7.

6. Ibid., 207–8.

7. Ibid., 210–11.

8. A. Keith, *Menders of the Maimed: The Anatomical & Physiological Principles Underlying the Treatment of Injuries to Muscles, Nerves, Bones, & Joints* (1919), 180.

9. A succinct sketch of Sayre's career is provided by his son, Reginald H. Sayre, in H. A. Kelly and W. L. Burrage, *Dictionary of American Medical Biography: Lives of Eminent Physicians of the United States and Canada, for the Earliest Times* (1928), 1079–80. The esteem in which his contemporaries held him comes through clearly in the eulogies written after his death. See, e.g., *Medical Record* (New York) *63* (1900): 505–6; *Boston Medical and Surgical Journal 163* (1900): 331; *Lancet 2* (1900): 1246. As a student, at the age of nineteen Sayre had already embarked on his public health crusade, issuing two pamphlets, *Cholera!!! Caution to*

the Public (New York Board of Health, n.d.), and *Directions to Prevent and Treat the Cholera* (1849). On the cholera scare of 1866 see C. E. Rosenberg, *The Cholera Years: The United States in 1832, 1849 and 1866* (1962), 175–225. See also I. M. Rutkow, *Surgery: An Illustrated History* (1993), 476–78.

10. Quoted in R. F. Stone, ed., *Biography of Eminent American Physicians and Surgeons*, 2d ed. (1898), 458.

11. "Circumcision versus Epilepsy, Etc.," *Medical Record* (New York) *5* (1870–71): 233–34.

12. L. A. Sayre, "Paralysis from Peripheral Irritation, So-Called 'Spinal Anaemia,'" *Medical and Surgical Reporter* (Philadelphia) *35* (1876): 305–8; R. Park, "Genital Irritation, Together with Some Remarks on the Hygiene of the Genital Organs in Young Children," *Chicago Journal and Examiner 41* (1880): 567.

13. L. A. Sayre, *On the Deleterious Results of a Narrow Prepuce and Preputial Adhesion* (1888). Lister's remark is quoted in H. Kelly and W. L. Burrage, *Dictionary of American Medical Biography*, 1080.

14. For an overview of reflex neurosis theory and "its breathtaking capacity to inspire meddlesomeness among doctors," see E. Shorter, *From Paralysis to Fatigue: A History of Psychosomatic Illness in the Modern Era* (1992), 20–24, 40–68, 86–94, quotation from p. 40.

15. Operations on women are the subject of G. J. Barker-Benfield, "Sexual Surgery in Late-Nineteenth-Century America," *International Journal of Health Services 5* (1975): 279–88, and idem, *Horrors of the Half-Known Life: Male Attitudes Toward Women and Sexuality in Nineteenth-Century America* (New York, 1976). Barker-Benfield contends that doctors' willingness to operate on women aggressively, indeed recklessly, stemmed from their anxiety about female emancipation. Surgery, he argues, was employed as a mechanism of social repression that, because it reflected a broad social unease, found ready acceptance among middle-class men and those in power. On Battey's operation see L. D. Longo, "The Rise and Fall in Battey's Operation: A Fashion in Surgery," *Bulletin of the History of Medicine 53* (1979): 224–67; and Shorter, *From Paralysis to Fatigue*, 75–78, quotation from p. 78.

16. A. Scull and D. Favreau, "The Clitoridectomy Craze," *Social Research 53* (1986), 243–60; idem, "'A Chance to Cut Is a Chance to Cure': Sexual Surgery for Psychosis in Three Nineteenth-Century Societies," in S. Spitzer and A. Scull, eds., *Research in Law, Deviance, and Social Control*, vol. 8 (1986), 3–39; Shorter, *From Paralysis to Fatigue*, 81–86.

17. G. M. Beard, "Nervous Diseases Connected with the Male Genital Function," *Medical Record* (New York) *22* (1882): 617–21, quotation from pp. 619–20.

18. E. E. Nichols, "Incontinence of Urine of Eight Years' Duration Relieved by Circumcision," *Medical Record* (New York) *15* (1879): 394; E. H. Richardson, Jr., "Congenital Phimosis and Adherent Prepuce Producing Anomalous Nervous Phenomena—Paralysis of Motion, and Dementia—Operation, Followed by Permanent Relief," *Transactions of the Medical Association of Georgia 31* (1880): 149; "Some of the Consequences of Phimosis and Adherent Prepuce," *Louisville Medical News 13* (1882): 25.

19. H. Horace Grant, "Phimosis the Cause of Convulsions in an Infant," *Medical Herald* (Louisville) *1* (1879–80): 223; E. P. Hurd, "Phimosis with Lithuria; Circumcision—Recov-

ery," *Medical and Surgical Reporter* (Philadelphia) *35* (1876): 395–97; J. A. Hofheimer, "Phimosis: A Plea for Its Relief by Early Operation," *Journal of the American Medical Association* *21* (1893): 890–91.

20. N. H. Chapman, "Some of the Nervous Affections Which Are Liable to Follow Neglected Congenital Phimosis in Children," *Medical News* (Philadelphia) *41* (1882): 317.

21. J. M. McGee, "Genital Irritation as a Cause of Nervous Disorders," *Mississippi Valley Medical Monthly 2* (1882): 103, quotes Gray's paper. While the popularity of reflex neurosis theory dwindled after the turn of the century, there were physicians who continued to fall back on it to justify circumcision. See E. J. Abbott, "Circumcision," *St. Paul Medical Journal* (Minnesota) *12* (1910): 71–74; C. F. Anderson, "Circumcision," *Journal of the Tennessee Medical Association 6* (1913–1914): 379–81; S. L. Kistler, "Rapid Bloodless Circumcision of Male and Female: Its Technic," *Journal of the American Medical Association 54* (1910): 1792.

22. McGee, "Genital Irritation," 103–5.

23. Norbert Elias, *The Civilizing Process,* trans. E. Jephcott, 2 vols. (1978); L. Wright, *Clean and Decent: The Fascinating History of the Bathroom and the Water Closet* (1960); H. D. Eberlein, "When Society First Took a Bath," in J. W. Leavitt and R. L. Numbers, eds., *Sickness and Health in America: Readings in the History of Medicine and Public Health* (1978), 335–38; R. L. Bushman, *The Refinement of America* (New York, 1993); S. Hoy, *Chasing Dirt: The American Pursuit of Cleanliness* (New York, 1995). For a succinct summary of this historiography, see R. L. Bushman, "Coming Clean," *The New Republic,* 3 July 1995, 39–41.

24. R. L. Bushman and C. L. Bushman, "The Early History of Cleanliness in America," *Journal of American History 74* (1988): 1213–38, quotation from p. 1214.

25. W. A. Alcott, "On Cleanliness," *The Moral Reformer and Teacher on the Human Constitution 1* (1835): 13, quoted in Bushman and Bushman, "Early History of Cleanliness," 1224.

26. Bushman and Bushman, "Early History of Cleanliness," 1230–31.

27. For a broadly allusive and insightful study of what germ theory meant to popular culture, see N. Tomes, *The Gospel of Germs: Men, Women, and the Microbe in American Life* (1998).

28. The collision of traditional empiricism with new bacteriological science is well described in N. Rogers, *Dirt and Disease: Polio Before FDR* (1992). The extent to which public health became more personalized toward the turn of the century and what a new focus on individuals and clinical practice meant are the subjects of a growing body of scholarship. The changing orientation of public health historiography may be followed in B. G. Rosenkrantz, *Public Health and the State: Changing Views in Massachusetts, 1842–1936* (1967); J. Duffy, *A History of Public Health in New York City,* 2 vols. (1968, 1974); idem, *The Sanitarians: A History of American Public Health* (1982); and J. W. Leavitt, *The Healthiest City: Milwaukee and the Politics of Health Reform* (1982). The more recent interest in how germ theory was popularized within the social context of public health is represented in N. Tomes, "The Private Side of Public Health: Sanitary Science, Domestic Hygiene, and the Germ Theory, 1870–1900," *Bulletin of the History of Medicine, 64* (1990): 509–39; B. Bates, *Bargaining for Life: A Social History of Tuberculosis* (1992); and J. W. Leavitt, "'Typhoid Mary' Strikes Back: Bacteriological Theory and Practice in Early Twentieth-Century Public Health," *Isis 83* (1992): 608–29.

29. C. V. Chapin, *How to Avoid Infection* (1917), 62; Leavitt, "'Typhoid Mary' Strikes Back," 621.

30. J. Y. Brown, "A Practical Suggestion in Regard to the Technique of the Operation of Circumcision," *Medical Mirror* (St. Louis) *1* (1890): 23.

31. P. C. Remondino, *History of Circumcision from the Earliest Times to the Present: Moral and Physical Reasons for Its Performance* (1891), 256, 11.

32. Remondino, *History of Circumcision*, 206–10, 255–56, 290–91, 300.

33. J. Ashurst, *The Principles and Practice of Surgery* (1878); H. Snow, *Clinical Notes on Cancer: Its Etiology and Treatment* (1883), 24; W. Rose and A. Carless, *A Manual of Surgery for Students and Practitioners* (1898), 1064.

34. For an account of General Grant's ordeal and "cancerphobia" in late Victorian America, see J. T. Patterson, *The Dread Disease: Cancer and Modern American Culture* (1987), 1–35; doctor's remark is from the *New York Tribune*, 31 July 1885, 27; Remondino, *History of Circumcision*, 227.

35. O. Temkin, "Therapeutic Trends and the Treatment of Syphilis Before 1900," *Bulletin of the History of Medicine 39* (1955): 309–16; A. M. Brandt, *No Magic Bullet: A Social History of Venereal Disease in the United States Since 1880*, expanded ed. (1987), 7–37.

36. Ashurst, *Principles and Practice of Surgery*, 945; Rose and Carless, *Manual of Surgery for Students and Practitioners*, 1064; S. Dunlop, "Case of Sebaceous Cysts of the Prepuce Resembling Epithelioma," *Medical Press* (London) *34* (1882), 372; D. B. Simmons, "A Case of Epileptiform Convulsion Cured by a Simple Detachment of a Glandulo-preputial Adhesion," *American Journal of Medical Science* (Philadelphia) *79* (1880), 444; E. von Bergmann, R. von Bruns, and J. von Mikulicz, *A System of Practical Surgery*, vol. 5. *Surgery of the Pelvis and Genito-Urinary Organs*, trans. W. T. Bull and E. M. Foote (1904), 627–30; A. C. Williams, "Circumcision," *Medical Standard* (Chicago) *6* (1889): 138–39; Simes, "Circumcision," 380. Remondino used the same logic: "The absence of the prepuce and the non-absorbing character of the skin of the glans penis, made so by constant exposure, with the necessary and unavoidably less tendency of these conditions to favor syphilitic inoculation" (*History of Circumcision*, 192).

37. J. S. Billings, "Vital Statistics of the Jews," *North American Review 152* (1891): 70–84; idem, *Vital Statistics of the Jews of the United States* (1890); H. M. Sachar, *A History of the Jews in America* (1992), 149.

38. A New York doctor, Abraham L. Wolbarst, conducted an extensive survey of his colleagues concerning differences in rates of several diseases between Jews and Gentiles. With a single exception, they reported sharply lower rates of venereal diseases and genital cancers among Jews. See Wolbarst, "Universal Circumcision as a Sanitary Measure," *Journal of the American Medical Association 62* (1914): 92–97.

39. This remark, which refers to the whole range of Jewish dietary and sanitary practices, is quoted in M. Fishberg, "Health and Sanitation of the Immigrant Jewish Population of New York," *Menorah 33* (1902): 73–82 (p. 75); Remondino, *History of Circumcision*, 186. Although an explanation of the difference remains elusive, researchers recently have confirmed that Jewish immigrants enjoyed substantially lower child mortality rates than non-Jews. See G. A. Condran and E. A. Kramarow, "Child Mortality Among Jewish Immigrants to the United States," *Journal of Interdisciplinary History 22* (1991): 223–54.

40. *Hebrew Observer*, 20 September 1867.

41. B. M. Ricketts, "One Hundred and Fifty Circumcisions," 364–65. Ricketts was not exaggerating, although the practice he described was comparatively rare. Wolbarst told his readers that he had "the assurance of Rabbi Philip Jaches of New York, who has successfully performed more than seven thousand circumcisions, that the ancient practice of sucking the wound is considered obsolete, and that cotton and gauze, wet with antiseptic solutions, are being commonly used for hemostasis." See Wolbarst, "Universal Circumcision as a Sanitary Measure," 93.

42. A. Brothers, "Gangrene of the Penis After Ritual Circumcision," *Medical Record* (New York) *51* (1897): 157; A. Schirman, "A Case of Tetanus in an Infant After Circumcision, with Recovery," *New York Medical Journal 62* (1895): 148; M. W. Ware, "A Case of Inoculation Tuberculosis After Circumcision," *New York Medical Journal 67* (1898): 287; C. H. Mastin, "Circumcision a Cause of Reflex Irritation of the Genito-Urinary Organs," *Gaillard's Medical Journal* (New York) *39* (1885): 355–62; F. C. Valentine, "Surgical Circumcision; Its Technique; Prevention of Infection; Its Legal Control," *Medical Record* (New York) *57* (1900): 1102–3; H. Levien, "Circumcision—Dangers of Unclean Surgery," *Medical Record* (New York), *46* (1894): 621.

43. R. Hochlerner, "Circumcision—Do We Need Legislation for It?" *Medical Record* (New York) *46* (1894): 702. Questions of technique and hygiene were raised in Germany and France; but physicians in those countries, intrigued by a new wave of comparative ethnography, continued to consider circumcision primarily as a religious ritual, not as a practice to be incorporated into the mainstream of medicine. See J. Jaffé, *Die rituelle Circumcision im Lichte der antiseptischen Chirurgie mit Berücksichtigung der religiösen Vorschriften* (1886); *Die Beschneidung in ihrer geschichtlichen, ethnographischen, religiösen und medicinischen Bedeutung . . .* , ed. A. Glassberg (1896); and J. B. Joly, *Histoire de la circoncision Étude critique du manuel opératoire des Musulmaus et des Israélites* (Paris, 1895).

44. N. M. Shaffer, "On Indiscriminate Circumcision," *Annals of the Anatomical and Surgical Society of Brooklyn 3* (1881), 243–47; H. Snow, *The Barbarity of Circumcision . . .* (1890); "Circumcision," *Medical Record* (New York) *46* (1894): 593.

45. R. Porter, *The Greatest Benefit to Mankind* (1998), 599.

46. Starr, *Social Transformation of American Medicine*, 164–70; C. E. Rosenberg, *The Care of Strangers: The Rise of America's Hospital System* (1987), 149.

47. M. S. Pernick, *A Calculus of Suffering: Pain, Professionalism, and Anesthesia in Nineteenth-Century America* (New York, 1985), 7, 237.

48. C. Knox-Shaw, "An Easy, Rapid, and Effectual Method of Performing Circumcision," *Homeopathic Journal of Obstetrics* (Philadelphia) *13* (1891): 209; G. W. Overall, "Painless Circumcision," *Medical Record* (New York) *39* (1891): 78. See also J. Madden, "Cocaine as an Anesthetic in Circumcision," *Therapeutic Gazette* (Detroit) *2* (1886): 229; and F. N. Otis, "Circumcision Under Cocaine," *New York Medical Journal, 43* (1886): 513.

49. S. E. Newman, "A Circumcision Operation for the Young," *Journal of the American Medical Association* 53 (1909): 1737; Brown, "A Practical Suggestion," 22; Simes, "Circumcision," 381–82.

50. S. Baruch, "New Circumcision Scissors," *Gaillard's Medical Journal* (New York) *33* (1882): 25–26; John W. Ross, "An Easy and Ready Method of Circumcision," *Medical Record*

(New York) *48* (1895): 323; A. U. Williams, "Circumcision," *Medical Standard* (Chicago) *6* (1889): 138. See also B. Lewis, "The Neatest Circumcision," *Medical Record* (St. Louis) *23* (1895): 81–83.

51. B. Merrill Ricketts, "Circumcision: The Last Fifty of Two Hundred Circumcisions," *New York Medical Journal 59* (1894): 431–32.

52. Hochlerner, "Circumcision," 702; Newman, "A Circumcision Operation for the Young," 1738.

53. Typical examples of the argument for operating as early as possible are W. B. Harlow's "Circumcision in Infancy," *Medical Record* (New York) *64* (1903): 495; and W. R. Wilson, "A Simple Method of Circumcision in the New-born," *Archives of Pediatrics 25* (1908): 841–43.

54. A. Jacobi, "On Masturbation and Hysteria in Young Children," *American Journal of Obstetrics 8* (1876): 595–606; S. H. Preston and M. R. Haines, *Fatal Years: Child Mortality in Late Nineteenth-Century America* (1991); S. Halpern, *Pediatrics: The Social Dynamics of Professionalism, 1880–1980* (1988), ch. 1; H. Levenstein, " 'Best for Babies' or 'Preventable Infanticide'? The Controversy over Artificial Feeding of Infants in America, 1880–1920," *Journal of American History 70* (1983): 76; R. A. Meckel, *Save the Babies: American Public Health Reform and the Prevention of Infant Mortality, 1850–1929* (1990), 40–61.

55. J. A. Hofheimer, "Phimosis: A Plea for Its Relief by Early Operation," *Journal of the American Medical Association 21* (1893): 890–91; H. L. Rosenberry, "Incontinence of Urine and Feces, Cured by Circumcision," *Medical Record* (New York): 173. In a cautionary response to Rosenberry's paper, John S. McCullough reported a case in which he recommended circumcision for a month-old baby with "severe indigestion." The parents refused and the boy died. See *Medical Record* (New York) *46* (1894): 342

56. J. W. Howe, *Excessive Venery, Masturbation, and Continence* (1896), 67; E. T. Brady, "Masturbation, with Illustrative Cases, and Remarks," *Virginia Medical Monthly 18* (1891–92): 259; F. P. Kinnicutt, "A Clinical Contribution on Insanity in Children, Induced by Masturbation," *Transactions of the American Neurological Association 1* (1875): 195–200. Although alienists and asylum doctors had linked masturbation to insanity since the early part of the nineteenth century, its great dangers were not a preoccupation of mainstream physicians until the 1860s. See E. H. Hare, "Masturbatory Insanity: The History of an Idea," *Journal of Mental Science 108* (1962): 1–20; and R. P. Neuman, "Masturbation, Madness, and the Modern Concepts of Childhood and Adolescence," *Journal of Social History 8* (1975): 1–27.

57. D. M. Feldman, *Birth Control in Jewish Law: Marital Relations, Contraception, and Abortion as Set Forth in the Classical Texts of Jewish Law* (1968), 114; L. M. Epstein, *Sex Laws and Customs in Judaism* (1967), 137; T. Szasz, "Routine Neonatal Circumcision: Symbol of the Birth of the Therapeutic State," *Journal of Medicine and Philosophy 21* (1996): 137–47.

58. R. Fowler, "What Are the Effects of Circumcision?" *Lancet 1* (1860): 382; R. Duchesne, "Effects of Circumcision," *Lancet 1* (1860): 412; T. Skinner, "Effects of Circumcision," *Lancet 1* (1860): 436; M. J. Moses, "The Value of Circumcision as a Hygienic and Therapeutic Measure," *New York Medical Journal 14* (1871): 368–74.

59. A. Johnson, "On an Injurious Habit Occasionally Met with in Infancy and Early Childhood," *Lancet 1* (1860): 344–45; J. Kellogg, *Treatment for Self-Abuse and Its Effects: Plain*

Facts for Young and Old (1888), 295; N. Bergman, "Report of a Few Cases of Circumcision," *Journal of Orificial Surgery* 7 (1889): 249–51.

60. D. Davis, "Housman's Hidden Perfections," *Times Literary Supplement*, 6 June 1998.

61. A. Money, *Treatment of Disease in Children* (1887), 421.

62. Remondino, *History of Circumcision*, 269; F. P. Kinnicutt, "A Clinical Contribution on Insanity in Children, Induced by Masturbation," *Transactions of the American Neurological Association 1* (1875): 195–200; The notion that masturbation in early childhood sets children on the path to destruction is given its fullest expression in Joseph Howe's *Excessive Venery, Masturbation and Continence* (1889). American society's enduring nervousness about childhood masturbation is documented in I. M. Marcus, ed., *Masturbation: From Infancy to Senescence* (New York, 1975).

63. R. N. Tooker, *All About Baby and Preparations for Its Advent . . .* (1896), 304; L. Emmett Holt, *The Diseases of Infancy and Childhood* (1902), 679–80; Remondino, *History of Circumcision*, 224.

64. Hurd, "Phimosis with Lithuria," 397 (italics in original).

65. A. J. Howe, *The Art and Science of Surgery* (Cincinnati, 1879), 691; S. W. Gross, *A Practical Treatise on Impotence, Sterility, and Allied Disorders of the Male Sexual Organs* (1890); Remondino, *History of Circumcision*, 216, 211; idem, "Some Observations on the History, Psychology, and Therapeutics of Impotence," *Pacific Medical Journal* 42 (1899): 522.

66. J. Hutchinson, "Our London Letter," *Medical News* 77 (1900): 707–8; E. Freeland, "Circumcision as a Preventive of Syphilis and Other Disorders," *Lancet 1* (1900): 1869–71.

67. Wolbarst, "Universal Circumcision as a Sanitary Measure," 92, 95. Examples of the quest for a reliable operation include J. A. Gardner and N. W. Wilson, "The Best Method of Infant Circumcision," *Buffalo Medical Journal* 41 (1901–1902): 891; H. J. Millstone, "A Cosmetically Perfect, Bloodless Circumcision," *Medical Record* (New York) *92* (1917): 680–82; C. T. Stone, "The Guillotine: A Simple One-Man Instrument for Doing Circumcisions," *Medical Record* (New York) *98* (1920): 479.

68. Remondino, *History of Circumcision*, iii. This physician-led movement, with its class-based view of the male body, is consistent with Charles Rosenberg's essay, "Sexuality, Class, and Role in Nineteenth-Century America," in C. Rosenberg, ed., *No Other Gods: On Science and American Social Thought* (1987).

69. M. Douglas, *Purity and Danger: An Analysis of Concepts of Pollution and Taboo* (1966), offers an interesting perspective on the sociocultural meanings of dirt and pollution in primitive societies. A suggestive treatment of the relationship between the role that images of dirt play in "fantasies of race" is J. Kovel, *White Racism: A Psychohistory* (1970), esp. 51–92.

70. Quoted in H. Kenner, "The Silent Minority," *New York Times Book Review*, 26 January 1997, 30.

71. Neonatal circumcision emerged at the same time physicians were broadly revising the practice of obstetrics, developing operations such as episiotomy (cutting the perineal tissues) to facilitate childbirth, and greatly expanding caesarean section deliveries. See J. W. Leavitt, *Brought to Bed: Childbearing in America, 1750–1950* (1986), esp. 142–70. The class dimension of the struggle between physicians and midwives is documented in N. S. Dye, "Modern Obstetrics and Working Class Women: The New Midwifery Dispensary, 1890–1920," *Journal of Social History*, 20 (1986–87): 549–64.

72. N. S. Dye and D. B. Smith, "Mother Love and Infant Death, 1750–1920," *Journal of American History* 73 (1986): 329–53, convincingly argue that through the early decades of the twentieth century, American mothers were responsive to medical advice that promised to help them evade the ravages of infant mortality. On the excessive modesty fostered by advice books, see R. Walters, *Primers for Prudery: Sexual Advice to Victorian America* (1974). F. G. Lydston, *Sex Hygiene for the Male* (1912), quoted in Wolbarst, "Universal Circumcision as a Sanitary Measure," 97.

73. M. Calnan, J. W. Douglas, and H. Goldstein, "Tonsillectomy and Circumcision: Comparisons of Two Cohorts," *International Journal of Epidemiology* 7 (1978): 78–85, confirms the hypothesis that both operations are correlated with social class, with better-off children receiving more surgery.

CHAPTER FIVE

1. T. Laqueur, *Making Sex: Body and Gender from the Greeks to Freud* (1990), 236; Soranus, *Gynecology*, trans. O. Temkin (1956), 14; G. Fallopio, *Observationes anatomica* (1565), 193. Fallopio's name is frequently cited in its Latin form, Fallopius.

2. C. Estienne, *De dissectione partium corporis humani* (1545), 289; L. Clendening, *Source Book of Medical History* (1942), 122.

3. F. L. Williams et al., eds., *Gray's Anatomy*, 3d ed. (1989), 1432.

4. J. Berengario da Carpi, *A Short Introduction to Anatomy (Isagogae Breves)*, trans. L. R. Lind (1959), 72–74; D. Jacquart and C. Thoimasset, *Sexuality and Medicine in the Middle Ages* (1988), 34.

5. G. Fallopio, "De praeputii brevitate corrigenda," *De decoratione* in *Opuscula* (1566), 49.

6. A. Paré, *Oeuvres Complétes: Revues et collationnées sur toutes les éditions avec les variantes*, vol. 2 (1970), 458–59.

7. W. Harvey, *The Anatomical Lectures of William Harvey (Prelectiones Anatomie Universalis De Musculis)*, ed. and trans. G. Whitteridge (1964), 213, 211.

8. D. Hart, "On the Role of the Epidermis in Forming Sheaths and Lumina to Organs, Illustrated Specially in the Development of the Prepuce and Urethra," *Journal of Anatomy* 42 (1907): 50; F. Jones, "The Development and Malformations of the Glans and Prepuce," *British Medical Journal* 1 (1910): 137; G. H. Edginton, "Embryological Significance of Certain Lesions of the Prepuce and Neighbourhood," *Glasgow Medical Journal* 74 (1910): 98.

9. G. Jefferson, "The Peripenic Muscle: Some Observations on the Anatomy of Phimosis," *Surgery, Gynecology, and Obstetrics* 23 (1916): 177–81.

10. H. C. Bazett, B. McGlone, R. G. Williams et al., "Depth, Distribution and Probable Identification in the Prepuce of Sensory End-Organs Concerned in Sensations of Temperature and Touch; Thermometric Conductivity," *Archives of Neurology and Psychiatry* 27 (1932): 489–517. This paper, with its labored discussion of spots on the prepuce sensitive to heat and cold, exemplifies the inconclusive, taxonomic approach taken by so many anatomists and pathologists during much of the twentieth century.

11. D. Gairdner, "The Fate of the Foreskin: A Study of Circumcision," *British Medical Journal* 2 (1949): 1433–37.

12. Ibid., 1434.

13. G. A. Deibert, "The Separation of the Prepuce in the Human Penis," *Anatomical Record 57* (1933): 389.

14. D. Gairdner, "The Fate of the Foreskin," 1434–35. Later (and larger) studies would confirm Gairdner's basic findings. See, e.g., H. Kayaba, H. Tamura, S. Kitajima et al., "Analysis of Shape and Retractabilty of the Prepuce in 603 Japanese Boys," *Journal of Urology 156* (1996): 1813–15.

15. Canadian Paediatric Association, Fetus and Newborn Committee, "Neonatal Circumcision Revisited," *Canadian Medical Association Journal 154* (1996): 769–80; N. Williams, J. Chell, L. Kapila, "Why Are Children Referred for Circumcision?" *British Medical Journal 306* (1993): 28; Kayaba, Tamura, Kitajima et al., "Analysis of Shape and Retractability," 1813–15.

16. Gairdner, "Fate of the Foreskin," 1436.

17. Ibid., 1437. Gairdner's findings were corroborated two decades later in a different population. See J. Oster, "Further Fate of the Foreskin: Incidence of Preputial Adhesions, Phimosis, and Smegma Among Danish Schoolboys," *Archives of Disease in Childhood* (1968): 200–202.

18. J. Smith, *Circumcision: A Guide to a Decision*, G. Francis, rev. and ed. (1979; 1993–1996), 2.

19. R. K. Winkelmann, "The Cutaneous Innervation of Human Newborn Prepuce," *Journal of Investigative Dermatology 26* (1956): 53–67; idem, "The Erogenous Zones: Their Nerve Supply and Significance," *Proceeding of the Staff Meetings of the Mayo Clinic 34* (1959): 39–47.

20. E. N. Preston, "Whither the Foreskin? A Consideration of Routine Neonatal Circumcision," *Journal of the American Medical Association 213* (1970): 1853–58.

21. A. Keith and A. Shellitoe, "The Preputial or Odiferous Glands of Man," *Lancet 1* (1904): 146; S. Parkash, S. Jeyakumar, K. Subramanyam et al., "Human Subpreputial Collection: Its Nature and Function," *Journal of Urology* (1973): 110–11; S. Prakash, R. Rao, K. Venkatesan et al., "Sub-Preputial Wetness—Its Nature," *Annals of National Medical Science 18* (1982): 109–12.

22. W. K. C. Morgan, "Penile Plunder," *Australian Medical Journal 1* (1967): 1102–3.

23. M. Maimonides, *Guide for the Perplexed*, vol. 3, trans. S. Pines (1974), 49; J. Bigelow, *The Joy of Uncircumcising* (1995), 22; T. J. Ritter, *Say No to Circumcision* (1992), 37.

24. P. M. Fleiss and F. Hodges, "The Foreskin Is Necessary," *Townsend Letter for Doctors and Patients* (April 1996): 2–3.

25. The anatomical discussion that follows is derived from J. R. Taylor, A. P. Lockwood, and A. J. Taylor, "The Prepuce: Specialized Mucosa of the Penis and Its Loss to Circumcision," *British Journal of Urology 77* (1996): 291–95.

26. The standard view in American medicine holds that sensation is focused in the glans. "The penis expands at its tip into the glans," writes Sherwin Nuland, "an acorn-shaped structure whose exquisite sensitivity is due to the vast numbers of nerve endings in its velvety-soft skin." See S. Nuland, *The Wisdom of the Body* (1997), 170.

27. J. R. Taylor, A. P. Lockwood, and A. J. Taylor, "The Prepuce," 291–95.

28. Ibid.

29. Advanced Tissue Sciences, *Annual Report 1995* (La Jolla, CA), 1–9; G. D. Gentzkow

et al., "Use of Dermagraft, a Cultured Human Dermis, to Treat Diabetic Foot Ulcers," *Diabetes Care 19* (1996): 350–54; "Circumcision Yielding Skin for Ulcerous Feet," *The Commercial Appeal* (Memphis), 7 May 1996; "Miracle Cures May Be in Your Cells," *Business Week*, 6 December 1993, 76–78; J. Pitta, "Biosynthetics," *Forbes*, 10 May 1993, 170–71.

CHAPTER SIX

1. M. S. Wilkes and S. Blum, "Current Trends in Routine Newborn Male Circumcision in New York State," *New York State Journal of Medicine 90* (1990): 243–46.

2. T. R. O'Brien, E. E. Calle, and W. K. Poole, "Incidence of Neonatal Circumcision in Atlanta, 1985–1986," *Southern Medical Journal 88* (1995): 411–18; E. E. Calle and M. J. Khoury, "Completeness of the Discharge Diagnoses as a Measure of Birth Defects Recorded in the Hospital Birth Record," *American Journal of Epidemiology 134* (1991): 69–77; J. B. Chessare, "Circumcision: Is the Risk of Urinary Tract Infection Really the Pivotal Issue?" *Clinical Pediatrics 31* (1992): 100–104.

3. In comparison, circumcision rates in most European countries were negligible. Canada, according to statistics compiled by provincial ministries of health, saw rates in 1996 drop from an earlier high of 46 percent to between 3 percent and 6 percent; Australia reported a rate of 10.6 percent for 1995–1996. The best indication of racial and ethnic distribution of circumcision is E. O. Lauman, C. M. Masi, and E. W. Zuckerman, "Circumcision in the United States," *Journal of the American Medical Association 277* (1997): 1052–57.

4. *Journal of the American Medical Association 185* (1963): 180; W. K. C. Morgan, "The Rape of the Phallus," *Journal of the American Medical Association 193* (1965): 124. Morgan's paper outraged many physicians, more for its attack on the legitimacy of circumcision than for its denigration of mothers, leading some to suggest that he deserved to be hauled before the House Un-American Activities Committee. See Morgan's "Reply to J. Greenblatt," *American Journal of Disease of Children 111* (April 1966): 448.

5. R. P. Bolande, "Ritualistic Surgery—Circumcision and Tonsillectomy," *New England Journal of Medicine 280* (1969): 591–96; American Child Health Association, *Physical Defects: The Pathway to Correction* (1934), ch. 8; J. E. Wennberg and J. P. Bunker, "The Need for Assessing Outcomes of Medical Practices," *Annual Review of Public Health 1* (1980): 277–95.

6. E. N. Preston, "Whither the Foreskin? A Consideration of Routine Neonatal Circumcision," *Journal of the American Medical Association 213* (1970): 1853–58. H. C. Thompson, L. R. King, E. Knox, and S. B. Korones, "Report of the Ad Hoc Task Force on Circumcision," *Pediatrics 56* (1975): 610–11. This study contained both a frank appraisal of the risks of the procedure and speculation that circumcision improved hygiene, and could help prevent and control sexually transmitted diseases and some cancers. B. Spock, Letter to the Editor, *Moneysworth*, 29 March 1976, 12.

7. D. A. Grimes, "Routine Circumcision of the Newborn Infant: A Reappraisal," *American Journal of Obstetrics and Gynecology 130* (1978): 125–29.

8. For a useful overview of the methodological problems in outcomes research, see J. S. Mandelblatt, D. G. Fryback, M. C. Weinstein et al., "Assessing the Effectiveness of Health

Interventions," in M. R. Gold, J. E. Siegel, L. B. Russell, M. C. Weinstein, eds., *Cost Effectiveness in Health and Medicine* (1996), 135–75.

9. M. Angell, *Science on Trial: The Clash of Medical Evidence and the Law in the Breast Implant Case* (1997), 97.

10. S. Blakeslee, "Placebos Prove So Powerful Even Experts Are Surprised," *New York Times*, 13 October 1998, D1, D4.

11. S. Blakeslee, "Enthusiasm of Doctor Can Give Pill Extra Kick," *New York Times*, 13 October 1998, D4.

12. A. Gawande, "When Doctors Make Mistakes," *The New Yorker*, 1 February 1999, 35.

13. S. L. Kistler, "Rapid Bloodless Circumcision," *Journal of the American Medical Association 54* (1910): 1782; J. B. Brimhall, "Gangrene Following Use of a Rubber Band in Surgery," *St. Paul Medical Journal 4* (1902): 490.

14. Canadian Paediatric Society, Fetus and Newborn Committee, "Neonatal Circumcision Revisited," *Canadian Medical Association Journal 154* (1996): 769–80; J. L. Snyderman, "The Problem of Circumcision in America," *The Truth Seeker*, July–August 1989, 39–42.

15. D. Gairdner, "The Fate of the Foreskin: A Study of Circumcision," *British Medical Journal 2* (1949): 1433–37.

16. H. Speert, "Circumcision of the Newborn: An Appraisal of the Present Status," *Obstetrics and Gynecology 2* (1953): 164–72.

17. W. F. Gee and J. S. Ansell, "Neonatal Circumcision: A Ten-Year Overview with Comparison of the Gomco Clamp and the Plastibell Device," *Pediatrics 58* (1976): 824–27; T. E. Wiswell and D. W. Geschke, "Risks from Circumcision During the First Month of Life Compared with Those for Uncircumcised Boys," *Pediatrics 83* (1989): 1011–15; U. Martinowitz, D. Varon, P. Jonas et al., "Circumcision in Hemophilia: The Use of Fibrin Glue for Local Hemostasis," *Journal of Urology 148* (1992): 855–57.

18. J. P. Gearhart and J. A. Rock, "Total Ablation of the Penis After Circumcision with Electrocautery," *Journal of Urology 142* (1989): 799–801.

19. "Family Gets $2.75 Million in Wrongful Surgery Suit," *Lake Charles American Press* (Louisiana), 28 May 1986; C. Seabrook, "Recent Accidents Involving Circumcision Renew Debate over Necessity of Procedure," *Atlanta Constitution*, 31 August 1985; "$22.8 Million in Botched Circumcision?" *Atlanta Constitution*, 12 March 1991; Gearhart and Rock, "Total Ablation of the Penis," 799–801.

20. J. A. Fraser, M. J. Allen, and P. F. Bagshaw, "A Randomised Trial to Assess Childhood Circumcision with the Plastibell Device Compared to a Conventional Dissection Technique," *British Journal of Surgery 68* (1981): 593–95; J. F. Redman and L. J. Schriber, "Postcircumcision Phimosis and Its Management," *Clinical Pediatrics 14* (1975): 407–9.

21. Fox Television News and Associated Press (New York), 30 November 1995.

22. N. Williams and L. Kapila, "Complications of Circumcision," *British Journal of Surgery 80* (1993): 1231–36; L. T. Byars and W. C. Trier, "Some Complications of Circumcision and Their Surgical Repair," *Archives of Surgery 76* (1958): 477–82; J. Shulman, N. Ben-Hur, and Z. Neuman, "Surgical Complications of Circumcision," *American Journal of the Diseases of Childhood 107* (1964): 149–54; M. Kon, "A Rare Complication of Circumcision: The Concealed Penis," *Journal of Urology 130* (1983): 573–74; J. Radhakrishnan and H. Reyes, "Penoplasty for Buried Penis Secondary to Radical Circumcision," *Journal of*

Pediatric Surgery 19 (1984): 629–31; G.W. Kaplan, "Complications of Circumcision," *Urologic Clinics of North America* 10 (1983): 543–49.

23. United States Patent and Trademark Office, "Disposable Circumcision Device," Appl. No. 218,548 (22 December 1980).

24. S. Isenberg and L. M. Elting, *Consumer's Guide to Successful Surgery* (1976), 271.

25. J. Lander, B. Brady-Freyer, J. B. Metcalfe et al., "Comparison of Ring Block, Dorsal Penile Nerve Block, and Topical Anesthesia for Neonatal Circumcision: A Randomized Controlled Trial," *Journal of the American Medical Association* 278 (1997): 2157–61.

26. K. J. Anand and P. R. Hickey, "Pain and Its Effects in the Human Neonate and Fetus," *New England Journal of Medicine* 317 (1987): 1321–29; P. Leach, *Babyhood* (1976).

27. American Academy of Pediatrics, Committee on the Fetus and Newborn, Committee on Drugs, Section on Anesthesiology, Section on Surgery, "Neonatal Anesthesia," *Pediatrics* 80 (1987): 446. The AAP reaffirmed this policy statement in favor of anesthesia in 1993.

28. F. Porter, "Pain in the Newborn," *Clinical Perinatology* 16 (1989): 549–64; F. L. Porter, R. H. Miller, and R. E. Marshall, "Neonatal Pain Cries: Effect of Circumcision on Acoustic Features and Perceived Urgency," *Child Development* 57 (1986): 790–802; H. J. Stang, M. R. Gunnar, L. Snellman et al., "Local Anesthesia for Neonatal Circumcision: Effects on Distress and Cortisol Response," *Journal of the American Medical Association* 259 (1988) 1507–11; H. H. Loughlin, N. E. Clapp Channing, S. H. Gelbach et al., "Early Termination of Breast Feeding: Identifying Those at Risk," *Pediatrics* 75 (1985): 508–13; N. Kurinij, P. H. Shiono, and G. G. Rhoads, "Breast-feeding Incidence and Duration in Black and White Women," *Pediatrics* 81 (1988): 365–71.

29. C. R. Howard, F. M. Howard, and M. L. Weitzman, "Acetaminophen Analgesia in Neonatal Circumcision: The Effect on Pain," *Pediatrics* 93 (1994): 641–46; J. Attia, C. Amiel-Tison, C. Mayer et al., "Measurement of Postoperative Pain and Narcotic Administration in Infants Using a New Clinical Scoring System," *Anesthesiology* 67 (1987): A532.

30. C. Kirya and M. W. Werthmann, Jr., "Neonatal Circumcision and Penile Dorsal Nerve Block—A Painless Procedure," *Journal of Pediatrics* 92 (1978): 998–1001; E. J. Schoen and A. A. Fischell, "Pain in Neonatal Circumcision," *Clinical Pediatrics* 30 (1991): 429–32; L. W. Snellman and H. J. Stang, "Prospective Evaluation of Complications of Dorsal Penile Nerve Block for Neonatal Circumcision," *Pediatrics* 95 (1995): 705–8; P. Fontaine, "Local Anesthesia for Neonatal Circumcision: Are Family Practice Residents Likely to Use It?" *Family Medicine* 22 (1990): 371–75; N. Wellington and M. J. Rieder, "Attitudes and Practices Regarding Analgesia for Newborn Circumcision," *Pediatrics* 92 (1993): 541–43.

31. Lander, Brady-Freyer, Metcalfe et al., "Comparison of Ring Block," 2157–62; A. Taddio, B. Stevens, K. Craig, et al., "Efficacy and Safety of Lidocaine-prilocaine Cream for Pain During Circumcision," *New England Journal of Medicine* 336 (1997): 1197–1201.

32. A. Taddio, B. Stevens, K. Craig et al., "Effect of Neonatal Circumcision on Pain Responses During Vaccination in Boys," *Lancet* 345 (1995): 291–92; A. Taddio, J. Katz, A. L. Ilersich, and G. Koren, "Effect of Neonatal Circumcision on Pain Response During Subsequent Routine Vaccination," *Lancet* 349 (1997): 599–603.

33. S. D. Niku, J. A. Stock, and G. W. Kaplan, "Neonatal Circumcision," *Urological Clinics of North America* 22 (1995): 57–65, quotation from pp. 58–59.

34. For a discussion of evaluative research, see J. E. Wennberg, "What Is Outcomes Research?" in A. C. Gelijns, ed., *Medical Innovation at the Crossroads*, vol. 1. *Modern Methods of Clinical Investigation* (1990), 33–46; and J. E. Wennberg, J. P. Bunker, and B. Barnes, "The Need for Assessing the Outcome of Common Medical Practices," *Annual Review of Public Health 1* (1980): 277–95.

35. D. M. Fergusson, J. M. Lawton, and F. T. Shannon, "Neonatal Circumcision and Penile Problems: An 8-Year Longitudinal Study," *Pediatrics 81* (1988): 537.

36. H. D. L. Birley et al., "Clinical Features and Management of Recurrent Balanitis: Association with Atopy and Genital Washing," *Genitourinary Medicine 69* (1993): 400–403; N. C. Kyuriazi and C. L. Costenbader, "Group A Beta-hemolytic Streptococcal Balanitis: It May Be More Common Than You Think," *Pediatrics 88* (1991): 154–56; N. Fakjian, S. Hunter, G. W. Cole, and J. Miller, "An Argument for Circumcision: Prevention of Balanitis in the Adult," *Archives of Dermatology 126* (1990): 1046–47.

37. W. S. Handley, *British Medical Journal 2* (1947): 841; E. L. Wynder, "A Study of Environmental Factors in Cancer of the Cervix," *American Journal of Obstetrics and Gynecology 68* (1954): 1046; E. L. Wynder and S. D. Licklider, "The Question of Circumcision," *Cancer 13* (1960): 442–45; S. I. McMillen, *None of These Diseases*, 2d ed. (1984), 91.

38. Approximately 85 percent of these cancers are squamous cell carcinomas, originating in the layer of tissue covering the outside of the cervix. Of the rest, most develop from gland cells (adenocarcinomas) or a combination of different cells. See I. Martinez, "Relationship of Squamous Cell Carcinoma of the Cervix Uteri to Squamous Cell Carcinoma of the Penis Among Puerto Rican Women Married to Men with Penile Carcinoma," *Cancer 24* (1969): 777–80; I. D. Rotkin, "Adolescent Coitus and Cervical Cancer: Associations of Related Events with Increased Risk," *Cancer Research 27* (1967): 603–17.

39. J. S. Wiener and P. J. Walther, "Human Papillomaviruses II: Association of HPV with GU Malignancies at Multiple Sites," *Infections in Urology 8* (1995): 165–70.

40. G. N. Weiss, "Prophylactic Neonatal Surgery and Infectious Diseases," *Journal of Pediatric Infectious Diseases 16* (1977): 727; see I. I. Kessler, "Etiological Concepts in Cervical Carcinogenesis," *Gynecological Oncology 12*, Suppl. 2 (1981): 7–24; W. C. Reeves, W. E. Rawls, and L. A. Brinton, "Epidemiology of Genital Papillomaviruses and Cervical Cancer," *Review of Infectious Diseases 11* (1989): 426–39; R. L. Poland, "The Question of Routine Neonatal Circumcision," *New England Journal of Medicine 322* (1990): 1314; E. Stern and P. Neely, "Cancer of the Cervix in Reference to Circumcision and Marital History," *Journal of the American Medical Women's Association 17* (1962): 739–40; Canadian Paediatric Society, Fetus and Newborn Committee, "Clinical Practice Guidelines," 769–80.

41. A. L. Wolbarst, "Circumcision and Penile Cancer," *Lancet 1* (1932): 150–53; A. L. Dean, *Journal of Urology 33* (1935): 252. Critics suggest that Wolbarst used the threat of penile cancer as a "scare tactic" in his crusade on behalf of circumcision. See P. M. Fleiss and F. Hodges, "Neonatal Circumcision Does Not Protect Against Cancer" (letter), *British Medical Journal 312* (1996): 779–80.

42. E. J. Schoen, "The Relationship Between Circumcision and Cancer of the Penis," *Journal of the American Cancer Society 41* (1991): 306–9.

43. C. J. Cold, M. R. Storms, and R. S. Van Howe, "Carcinoma in Situ of the Penis in a 76-Year-Old Circumcised Man," *Journal of Family Practice 44* (1997): 407–9; N. K. Bissada,

"Post-Circumcision Carcinoma of the Penis: Clinical Aspects," *Journal of Urology 135* (1986): 283–85.

44. M. Kochen and S. McCurdy, "Circumcision and the Risk of Cancer of the Penis: A Life-Table Analysis," *American Journal of Diseases in Childhood 134* (1980): 484–86; L. Garfinkel, "Circumcision and Penile Cancer" (letter), *California Cancer Journal Clinic 33* (1983): 320; S. J. Culture and J. L. Young, eds., *Third National Cancer Survey Incidence Data,* Monograph 41, National Cancer Institute (1975); J. L. Young, C. L. Percy, and A. J. Asire, eds., *Surveillance, Epidemiology, and End Results Incidence and Mortality Data 1973–1977,* Monograph 57, National Cancer Institute (1981); P. A. Wingo, T. Tong, and S. Bolden, "Cancer Statistics," *California Cancer Journal Clinic 45* (1995): 8–30; T. E. Wiswell, "Neonatal Circumcision: A Current Appraisal," *Focus and Opinion: Pediatrics 1* (1995):

45. M. Frisch, S. Friis, S. K. Kjaer et al., "Falling Incidence of Penis Cancer in an Uncircumcised Population—Denmark, 1943–1990," *British Medical Journal 311* (1995): 1471.

46. J. W. Duckett, "A Temperate Approach to Neonatal Circumcision," *Urology 46* (1995): 771–72.

47. L. A. Brinton, J. Y. Li, S. D. Rong et al., "History of Circumcision, Medical Conditions, and Sexual Activity and Risk of Penile Cancer," *International Journal of Cancer 85* (1993): 19–24; G. A. Magoha and R. F. Kaale, "Epidemiological and Clinical Aspects of Carcinoma of the Penis at Kenyatta National Hospital," *East Africa Medical Journal 72* (1995): 359–61.

48. C. Maden, K. J. Sherman, A. M. Beckmann et al., "History of Circumcision, Medical Conditions, and Sexual Activity and Risk of Penile Cancer," *JNCI 85* (1993): 19–24.

49. H. Shingleton and C. W. Heath, Jr. (American Cancer Society) to Peter Rappo (American Academy of Pediatrics), 16 February 1996; D. Cadman, A. Gafni, and J. McNamee, "Newborn Circumcision: An Economic Perspective," *Journal of the Canadian Medical Association 131* (1984): 1353–55.

50. C. Quétel, *History of Syphilis,* trans. J. Braddock and B. Pike (1990), 56.

51. *Newsweek,* 21 July 1947, 49; E. A. Hand, "Circumcision and Venereal Disease," *Archives of Dermatology and Syphilis 60* (1949): 341–46; R. A. Wilson, "Circumcision and Venereal Disease," *Canadian Medical Association Journal, 56* (1947): 54–56; Gairdner, "Fate of the Foreskin," 1436.

52. S. W. Parker, A. J. Stewart, M. N. Wren et al., "Circumcision and Sexually Transmissible Disease," *Medical Journal of Australia 2* (1983): 288–90; C. Maden, K. J. Sherman, A. M. Beckmann et al., "History of Circumcision, Medical Conditions, and Sexual Activity and Risk of Penile Cancer," *Journal of the National Cancer Institute 85* (1993): 19–24.

53. L. S. Cook, L. A. Koutsky, and K. K. Holmes, "Circumcision and Sexually Transmitted Diseases," *AJPH 84* (1995): 197–201; Parker, Stewart, Wren et al., "Circumcision and Sexually Transmissible Disease," 288–90.

54. S. Prakash, R. Rao, K. Venkatesan, and S. Ramakrishnan, "Sub-preputial Wetness—Its Nature," *Annals of the National Medical Society* (India) *18* (1982): 109–12; M. R. Storms, unpublished letter, *Circumcision* (online journal) *2* (1997): http://faculty.washington. edu/ged/CIRCUMCISION*weber.u.washington.edu/~gcd/circumcision/v2n1.html.*

55. Cook, Koutsky, and Holmes, "Circumcision and Sexually Transmitted Diseases," 200.

56. The 1992 NHSLS includes 1,511 men and 1,981 women between the ages of eighteen and fifty-nine who live in households, representative of an estimated 97 percent of the United States population. It does not cover the homeless or people who live in group facilities such as prisons, military barracks, or college dormitories. The basic questionnaire was administered in a face-to-face interview, lasting an average of ninety minutes.

57. E. O. Laumann, C. M. Masi, and E. W. Zuckerman, "Circumcision in the United States: Prevalence, Prophylactic Effects, and Sexual Practice," *Journal of the American Medical Association* 277 (1997): 1052–57. The results of the National Health and Social Life Survey have been published in two books: R. T. Michael, J. H. Gagnon, E. O. Laumann, and G. Kolata, *Sex in America: A Definitive Survey* (1995), and E. O. Laumann, J. H. Gagnon, R. T. Michael, and S. Michaels, *The Social Organization of Sexuality in the United States* (1994).

58. Laumann, Masi, and Zuckerman, "Circumcision in the United States," 1052–57. Unsurprisingly, the conclusion that removing the foreskin doesn't protect men from STDs led circumcision advocates to attack Laumann's research methods. For example, Edgar J. Schoen, who served as chairman of the 1988 American Academy of Pediatrics Task Force on Circumcision and has remained a vocal defender of neonatal circumcision, insisted that because the NHSLS survey depended on self-reported cases of STDs, its data were unreliable; see E. J. Schoen, "Letters," *Journal of the American Medical Association* 278 (1997): 201. The authors replied that their study acknowledged the problems of underreporting, but "lacking a plausible mechanism that links the presence or absence of a foreskin with a differential ability to recall and report medically diagnosed STD experiences, we fail to see the significance of Schoen's remarks regarding our findings." See E. O. Laumann, C. M. Masi, and E. W. Zuckerman, "Letters," *Journal of the American Medical Association* 278 (1997): 203.

59. "Evidence That Circumcision Reduces Susceptibility to HIV Infection Called Substantial," Reuters wire service report, 10 July 1996.

60. J. C. Caldwell and P. Caldwell, "The African AIDS Epidemic," *Scientific American* 274 (1996): 62–68.

61. A. Nicoll, "Routine Male Circumcision and Risk of Infection with HIV–1 and Other Sexually Transmitted Diseases," *Archives of Disease in Childhood* 77 (1997): 194–95.

62. V. R. Staiman, D. J. Kwan, and F. C. Lowe, "Genitourinary Manifestation of AIDS," *Infections in Urology* 9 (1996): 73–78, 92; R. A. Royce, A. Sena, W. Cates, Jr. et al., "Sexual Transmission of HIV," *New England Journal of Medicine* 336 (1997): 1072–78.

63. M. Sassan-Morokro, A. E. Greenberg, I. M. Coulibaly et al., "High Rates of Sexual Contact with Female Sex Workers, Sexually Transmitted Diseases, and Condom Neglect Among HIV-Infected and Uninfected Men with Tuberculosis in Abijan, Côte d'Ivoire," *Journal of Acquired Immune Deficiency Syndrome and Human Retrovirology* 11 (1996): 183–87. For a discussion of the methodological problems, see I. De Vincenzi and T. Mertens, "Male Circumcision: A Role in HIV Prevention?" *AIDS* 8 (1994): 153–60.

64. H. Grosskurth, F. Mosha, J. Todd et al., "A Community Trial of the Impact of Improved Sexually Transmitted Disease Treatment on the HIV Epidemic in Rural Tanzania: 2 Baseline Survey Results," *AIDS* 9 (1995): 927–34; M. Guimares, E. Castiho, C. Ramos-Filho et al., "Heterosexual Transmission of HIV-I: A Multicenter Study in Rio de Janeiro, Brazil," Seventh International Conference on AIDS, Florence, Italy, June 1991.

65. E. Schoen, "Circumcision Updated—Implicated?" *Pediatrics* 92 (1993): 388–91.

66. T. E. Wiswell, F. R. Smith, and J. W. Bass, "Decreased Incidence of Urinary Tract Infections in Circumcised Male Infants," *Pediatrics* 75 (1985): 901–3; T. E. Wiswell and J. D. Roscelli, "Corroborative Evidence for the Decreased Incidence of Urinary Tract Infections in Circumcised Male Infants," *Pediatrics* 78 (1986): 96–99.

67. C. M. Ginsburg and G. H. McCracken, Jr., "Urinary Tract Infection in Young Infants," *Pediatrics* 69 (1982): 409–12; Wiswell and Roscelli, "Corroborative Evidence," 96–99; U. B. Berg, "Renal Dysfunction in Recurrent Urinary Tract Infections in Childhood," *Pediatric Nephrology* 3 (1989): 9–15; H. G. Rushton, "Pyelonephritis in Male Infants: How Important Is the Foreskin?" *Journal of Urology* 148 (1992): 733–36; T. E. Wiswell et al., "Declining Frequency of Circumcision: Implications for Changes in the Absolute Incidence and Male to Female Sex Ratio of Urinary Tract Infections in Early Infancy," *Pediatrics* 79 (1987): 331–48; T. E. Wiswell et al., "Effects of Circumcision Status on Periurethral Bacterial Flora During the First Year of Life," *Journal of Pediatrics* 113 (1988): 442–46; T. E. Wiswell and W. E. Hachey, "Urinary Tract Infections and the Uncircumcised State: An Update," *Clinical Pediatrics* 32 (1993): 130–34.

68. The linchpin of any argument about health differences between circumcised and uncircumcised populations is to distinguish one from the other. But in very large studies based on medical records this is hard to do, because the record keeping is so sloppy. See O'Brien, Calle, and Poole, "Incidence of Neonatal Circumcision in Atlanta," 411–18. J. C. Craig, J. F. Knight, P. Sureshkumar et al., "Effects of Circumcision on Incidence of Urinary Tract Infection in Preschool Boys," *Journal of Pediatrics* 128 (1996): 23–27; American Academy of Pediatrics, Task Force on Circumcision, "Circumcision Policy Statement (RE9850)," *Pediatrics* 103 (1999): 686–93.

69. R. H. Epstein, "Circumcision Controversy: Doctors Debate the Benefits and Risks of This Common Procedure, but for Most Parents the Decision Is Personal," *Washington Post*, 7 October 1997, Z14.

70. J. A. Roberts, "Neonatal Circumcision: An End to the Controversy?" *Southern Medical Journal* 89 (1996): 167–71.

71. Craig, Knight, Sureshkumar et al., "Effect of Circumcision on Incidence of Urinary Tract Infection," 23–27; H. A. Cohen, M. M. Drucker, S. Vanier et al., "Postcircumcision Urinary Tract Infection," *Clinical Pediatrics* 31 (1992): 322–24. Additional research has corroborated the association between *berit milah* and UTI. "We conclude that the high incidence of UTI following a ritual Jewish circumcision, as well as the relatively high preponderance of bacteria other than *E. coli*, may suggest a causal relationship between circumcision and UTI," wrote M. Goldman, J. Barr, T. Bistritzer et al., "Urinary Tract Infection Following Ritual Jewish Circumcision," *Israeli Journal of Medical Science* 32 (1996): 1098–1102. For research suggesting some benefit for older males, see D. H. Sprach et al., "Lack of Circumcision Increases the Risk of Urinary Tract Infections in Young Men," *Journal of the American Medical Association* 267 (1992): 679–81.

72. C. K. Mitchell, S. M. Franco, and R. L. Vogel, "Incidence of Urinary Tract Infections in an Inner-City Outpatient Population," *Journal of Perinatology* 15 (1995): 131–34; L. Pead and R. Maskell, "Study of Urinary Tract Infection in Children in One Health District," *British Medical Journal* 309 (1994): 631–34; E. K. Hamburger, "Urinary Tract Infections in Infants and Children: Guidelines for Averting Permanent Damage," *Postgraduate Medicine* 80 (1986): 235–38, 240–41; U. Jodal, "The Natural History of Bacteriuria in Childhood," *In-*

fectious Diseases Clinics of North America 1 (1987): 713–29; M. Chandra, "Reflux Nephropathy, Urinary Tract Infection, and Voiding Disorders," *Current Opinion in Pediatrics 7* (1995): 164–70.

73. F. E. Gareau, D. C. Mackel, J. R. Borning, III et al., "The Acquisition of Fecal Flora by Infants from Their Mothers During Birth," *Journal of Pediatrics 54* (1959): 313–18; J. F. Kenny, D. N. Medearis, Jr., S. W. Klein et al., "An Outbreak of Urinary Tract and Other Infections Due to *E. coli*," *Pediatrics 33* (1964): 865–71; K. Tullus, K. Horlin, S. B. Svenson et al., "Epidemic Outbreaks of Acute Pyelonephritis Caused by Nosocomial Spread of P-fimbriated *Escherichia coli* in Children," *Journal of Infectious Diseases 150* (1984): 728–36.

74. E. N. Fussell, M. B. Knaack, R. Cherry et al., "Adherence of Bacteria to Human Foreskins," *Journal of Urology 140* (1988): 997–1001; G. Kallenius, R. Mollby, S. B. Svenson et al., "Occurrence of P-fimbriated *Escherichia coli* in Urinary Tract Infections," *Lancet 2* (1981): 1366–69; J. A. Roberts, "Does Circumcision Prevent Urinary Tract Infection?" *Journal of Urology 135* (1986): 991; idem, "Etiology and Pathophysiology of Pyelonephritis," *American Journal of Kidney Disease 17* (1991): 1–9.

75. F. U. Eke and N. N. Eke, "Renal Disorders in Children: A Nigerian Study," *Pediatric Nephrology 8* (1994): 383–86; Pead and Maskell, "Study of Urinary Tract Infection in Children," 631–34; J. M. Smellie and S. P. Rigden, "Pitfalls in the Investigation of Children with Urinary Tract Infection," *Archives of the Diseases of Childhood 72* (1995): 251–55 (see also pp. 255–58); Mitchell, Franco, and Vogel, "Incidence of Urinary Tract Infection," 131–34; L. M. Shortliffe, "The Management of Urinary Tract Infections in Children Without Urinary Tract Abnormalities," *Urologic Clinics of North America 22* (1995): 67–73; S. Hellerstein, "Urinary Tract Infections: Old and New Concepts," *Pediatric Clinics of North America 42* (1995): 1433–57; American Academy of Pediatrics, Task Force on Circumcision, "Circumcision Policy Statement," 686–93.

76. Williams and Kapila, "Complications of Circumcision," 1231–36; Wiswell and Geschke, "Risks from Circumcision," 1011–15.

77. Canadian Paediatric Society, Fetus and Newborn Committee, "Neonatal Circumcision Revisited," 769–80; R. S. Thompson, "Is Routine Circumcision Indicated in the Newborn? An Opposing View," *Journal of Family Practice 31* (1990): 189–97.

78. F. H. Lawler, R. S. Bisonni, and D. R. Holtgrave, "Circumcision: A Decision Analysis of Its Medical Value," *Family Medicine 23* (1991): 587–93; T. G. Ganiats, J. B. C. Humphrey, H. L. Taras et al., "Routine Neonatal Circumcision: A Cost-Utility Analysis," *Medical Decision Making 11* (1991): 282–93.

79. Laumann, Masi, and Zuckerman, "Circumcision in the United States," 1052–57.

80. Ibid., 1055–56; L. Leibovich, "(Circumcised) Boys Just Want to Have Fun," *Daily Clicks: Newsreal*, 25 March 1998.

81. See, e.g., E. J. Schoen, "Circumcision in the United States: Prevalence, Prophylactic Effects, and Sexual Practice," letter, *Journal of the American Medical Association 278* (1997): 200; I. R. Berman, "Circumcision in the United States: Prevalence, Prophylactic Effects, and Sexual Practice," letter, *Journal of the American Medical Association 278* (1997): 200.

CHAPTER SEVEN

1. "Declaration of the First International Symposium on Circumcision," 3 March 1989, Anaheim, CA.

2. M. Milos, "Infant Circumcision: 'What I Wish I Had Known'" (1988): *www.cirp.org/CIRP/pages/riley/wish.*

3. Quoted in J. Bigelow, *The Joy of Uncircumcising!* 2d ed. (1995), 127.

4. M. Milos and D. Macris, "Circumcision: A Medical or Human Rights Issue?" *Journal of Nurse-Midwifery* (1992).

5. John P. Warren et al., "Circumcision of Children" (letter), *British Medical Journal 312* (1996): 377.

6. J. A. Erickson, *Deeper into Circumcision: An Invitation to Awareness*, Chicago ed. (1996), 61.

7. A. Zavales, *The International Human Rights Challenge of Genital Mutilation & the United Nations: Initiating a Global Dialogue on the Transcultural, Multireligious, & Interdisciplinary Dimensions of Appropriating Universal Human Rights Paradigms* (1994), 49n34.

8. For a historical account of American medical ethics, see D. Rothman, *Strangers at the Bedside: A History of How Law and Bioethics Transformed Medical Decision Making* (1992).

9. The documentary film was Barry Ellworth's *The Nurses of St. Vincent: Saying "No" to Circumcision* (1993).

10. M. Milos to author, personal communication, 9 May 1999.

11. American Academy of Pediatrics, Committee on Fetus and Newborn, *Standards and Recommendations for Hospital Care of Newborn Infants*, 5th ed. (1971), 110.

12. H. Thompson, L. King, E. Knox et al., "Report of the Ad Hoc Task Force on Circumcision," *Pediatrics 56* (1975), 610–11.

13. Ibid., 611.

14. American Academy of Pediatrics, Committee on Fetus and Newborn, *Guidelines for Perinatal Care* (1983).

15. "Donahue," transcript no. Q6177 (1987).

16. "ABC News Nightline," show no. 1879 (1988).

17. Ultimately, in 1988, the CMA's scientific advisory board, unable to find credible evidence for Dr. Fink's claims that circumcision helped prevent sexually transmitted diseases, including AIDS, decided to table the issue.

18. E. J. Schoen, "Ode to the Circumcised Male," *American Journal of Diseases in Children 141* (1987): 128.

19. American Academy of Pediatrics, "Report of the Task Force on Circumcision," *Pediatrics 84* (1989): 388–91.

20. J. Trager, "Forget Those Headlines About Circumcision: AAP Is Against Routine Circumcision," *Medical Tribune 30* (1989): 16.

21. PBS, "MacNeil-Lehrer New Hour," 27 March 1989.

22. American Academy of Pediatrics, Task Force on Circumcision, "Circumcision Policy Statement," *Pediatrics 103* (1999): 686–93.

23. J. E. Brody, "Circumcision, Yes or No? A Guide for Perplexed Parents," *New York Times*, 16 March 1999 (online version), 1; see also D. Stead, "Circumcision's Pain and Benefits Re-Examined, *New York Times*, 2 March 1999 (online version), 1–3.

24. See *Circumcision* 1 (1996) at http://faculty.washington.edu/gced/CIRCUMCISION Brady, "Low-Ranking Soldier" (letter), *Circumcision* 2 (1997): 8. The online journal is also linked through NOCIRC's Internet homepage.

25. Two accessible reviews of this controversy are P. Hartge, "Abortion, Breast Cancer, and Epidemiology," *New England Journal of Medicine 336* (1997): 127–28, and M. Gammon, J. Bertin, and M. Terry, "Abortion and the Risk of Breast Cancer: Is There a Believable Association?" *Journal of the American Medical Association 275* (1996): 24–31.

26. National Right to Life Council's web site is *www.prolife.org*.

27. R. Goldman, *Circumcision: The Hidden Trauma* (1997), 168.

28. J. Hutchinson, "Our London Letter," *Medical News 77* (1900): 707–8.

29. C. W. Cockshut, "Circumcision," *British Medical Journal 2* (1935): 764.

30. Bigelow, *Joy of Uncircumcising!*, 112. Some historical context is given in S. L. Gilman, "Decircumcision: The First Aesthetic Surgery," *Modern Judaism 17* (1997): 201–301.

31. J. Penn, "Penile Reform," *British Journal of Plastic Surgery 16* (1963): 287.

32. N. R. Feins, "A New Incision for Penile Surgery," *Journal of Pediatric Surgery 16* (1981): 817–19; D. M. Greer et al., "A Technique for Foreskin Restoration and Some Preliminary Results," *Journal of Sex Research 18* (1982): 324–30.

33. "Donahue," transcript no. Q6177 (1987).

34. Bigelow, *Joy of Uncircumcising*, 128–29.

35. National Organization of Restoring Men (NORM), "Governing Policies" (n.d.).

36. T. Hammond, "Awakenings: A Preliminary Poll of Circumcised Men (Revealing the Long-Term Harm and Healing the Wounds of Infant Circumcision), Report of the Harm Documentation Survey (1994).

37. Bigelow, *Joy of Uncircumcising*, 115.

38. Quoted in Erickson, *Deeper into Circumcision*, 126–27; T. Pong, "Circumcision: The Pain and Trauma," autobiographical sketch (1993), quoted in Goldman, *Circumcision: The Hidden Trauma*, 97.

39. D. Chamberlain, "Babies Remember Pain," *Pre and Perinatal Psychology Journal 3* (1989): 304.

40. J. Money and J. Davidson, "Adult Penile Circumcision: Erotosexual and Cosmetic Sequelae," *Journal of Sex Research 19* (1983): 289–92.

41. "Circumcision: What You Think," *Australian Forum 11* (1989): 10–29; "Circumcision Uncut," *Men's Confidential* (March 1996): 10–11; T. Hammond, "A Preliminary Poll of Men Circumcised in Infancy or Childhood," *British Journal of Urology 83*, Suppl. 1 (1999): 85–92.

42. P. Toussieng, "Men's Fear of Having Too Small a Penis," *Medical Aspects of Human Sexuality 11* (1977): 62–70.

43. Cosmetic Surgery International, "The Procedures," Reed Centre, "Penile Enlargement," *www.enlargepenis.com*.

44. Bigelow, *Joy of Uncircumcising*, 138, 132.

45. Ibid., 169–70.

46. Ibid., 135–36.

47. Ibid., 143.

CHAPTER EIGHT

1. A. M. Rosenthal, "To the Clintons and the Doles," *New York Times*, 28 May 1996; idem, "Fighting Female Mutilation," *New York Times*, 12 April 1996.

2. C. W. Dugger, "Woman, Seeking Asylum, Endures Prison in America," *New York Times*, 15 April 1996.

3. C. W. Dugger, "U.S. Grants Asylum to Woman Fleeing Genital Mutilation Rite," *New York Times*, 14 June 1996.

4. M. Simons, "Eight-Year Sentence in France for Genital Cutting," *New York Times*, 18 February 1999, A3.

5. C. W. Dugger, "Genital Cutting in Africa: Slow to Challenge an Ancient Ritual," *New York Times*, 5 October 1995 (www); F. Bryk, *Circumcision in Man and Woman: Its History, Psychology and Ethnology*, trans. D. Berger (1934), 270.

6. O. Dapper, *Beschreibung von Afrika* (1670), 102.

7. J. Lantier, *La Cite Magique et Magie en Afrique Noire* (1972), trans. F. Hosken; *Munger Africana Library Notes 36* (1976): 11.

8. I. A. Mansurnoor, *Islam in an Indonesian World* (1990), 71–72; N. el-Saadawi, *The Hidden Face of Eve: Women in the Arab World*, trans. and ed. S. Hetata (1980), 36–40.

9. Quoted in D. Jacquart and C. Thomasset, *Sexuality and Medicine in the Middle Ages* (1988), 34.

10. R. Burton, *The Book of the Thousand Nights and a Night* (1885), 279.

11. Quoted in S. A. abu-Sahlieh, *To Mutilate in the Name of Jehovah or Allah: Legitimization of Male and Female Circumcision* (1994), 6.

12. Ibid., 10.

13. Ibid., 15.

14. El-Saadawi, *Hidden Face of Eve*, 33.

15. World Health Organization, Khartoum Seminar on Traditional Practices Affecting the Health of Women and Children, Khartoum, Sudan, 1979.

16. N. Toubia, "Female Circumcision as a Public Health Issue," *New England Journal of Medicine 331* (1994): 712–16; World Health Organization, *Female Genital Mutilation* (1997).

17. After the CNN broadcast, the Egyptian government sued CNN for $500, alleging that the circumcision footage damaged Egypt's reputation. The courts subsequently threw out the suit. United Nations, *Report of the International Conference on Population and Development* (1994); United Nations, *Report of the Fourth World Conference on Women* (1995).

18. D. Jehl, "Egyptian Court Overturns Ban on Cutting of Girls' Genitals," *New York Times*, 26 June 1997, A9.

19. M. A. Anees, "Genital Mutilations: Moral or Misogynous?" *Islamic Quarterly 33* (1989): 101–17.

20. Nemesius of Emesa, *On the Nature of Man*, ed. W. Tefler (1955), 369.

21. W. Laqueur, *Making Sex: Body and Gender from Greeks to Freud* (1990), 4; F. Netter, *Atlas of Human Anatomy*, 2d ed. (1997), plate 350.

22. C. Niebuhr, *Beschreibung von Arabien* (1772); H. Ploss, *Das Weib in Natur- und Voelkerkunde* (1887), quoted in Bryk, *Circumcision in Man and Woman*, 286–87.

23. See www.rjglib.carn/thoughts/circumcision/response.html.

24. Quoted in L. Burstyn, "Female Circumcision Comes to America," *Atlantic Monthly* 276 (1996): 29. For a balanced discussion of the issue, see S. A. James, "Reconciling International Human Rights and Cultural Relativism: The Case of Female Circumcision," *Bioethics 8* (1994): 1–26; and L. M. Kopelman, "Female Circumcision/Genital Mutilation and Ethical Relativism," *Second Opinion 20* (1994): 55–71.

25. The U.S. law was added to Sections 664 and 665 of the Illegal Immigration Reform and Immigrant Responsibility Act of 1996, Division C, *Omnibus Consolidated Appropriations Act for Fiscal 1997,* Public Law no. 104–208, 30 September 1996; American College of Obstetricians and Gynecologists, *Committee Opinion: Female Genital Mutilation* (1995), 151; Council on Scientific Affairs, "Female Genital Mutilation," *Journal of the American Medical Association 274* (1995): 1714–16; American Academy of Pediatrics, Committee on Bioethics, "Female Genital Mutilation (RE9749)," *Pediatrics 102* (1998): 153–56.

26. The tenacity of these practices is described in L. Williams and T. Sobieszczyk, "Attitudes Surrounding the Continuation of Female Circumcision in the Sudan: Passing Tradition to the Next Generation," *Journal of Marriage and the Family 59* (1997): 966–82.

27. B. Crossette, "Senegal Bans Cutting of Genital of Girls," *New York Times*, 18 January 1999, A7; D. Hecht, "Female Circumcision," National Public Radio, "All Things Considered," 28 July 1998.

28. S. I. Kistler, "Rapid Bloodless Circumcision," *Journal of the American Medical Association 54* (1910): 1782; R. Porter, *The Greatest Benefit to Mankind* (1998), 364.

29. W. G. Rathmann, "Female Circumcision: Indications and a New Technique," *General Practitioner 20* (1959): 115–20; R. Gross et al., "Clitoredectomy for Sexual Abnormalities," *Surgery 59* (1966): 300–308.

30. C. Kellison, "Circumcision for Women—The Kindest Cut of All," *Playgirl* (October 1973), 76; J. F. Perlmutter, Letter, *Medical Aspects of Human Sexuality 10* (1976): 143; National Blue Shield Association, Press Release, 18 May 1977.

31. N. Angier, "In a Culture of Hysterectomies, Many Question Their Necessity," *New York Times*, 17 February 1997, A1, 10.

32. Quoted in N. Angier, "New Debate over Surgery on Genitals," *New York Times*, 13 May 1997, C6.

33. J. Colapinto, "The True story of John/Joan," *Rolling Stone*, 11 December 1997, 92–96.

34. "Is Early Vaginal Reconstruction Wrong for Some Intersex Girls?" *Urology Times*, February 1997, 10–12; quoted in Angier, "New Debate over Surgery on Genitals," C6.

35. W. G. Reiner, "Sex Assignment in the Neonate with Intersex of Inadequate Genitalia," *Archives of Pediatric and Adolescent Medicine 151* (1997): 1044–45.

36. L. Kamps, "Labia Envy," *Salon @ www.salonmagazine.com/mwt/feature/1998/03/16feature.html.*

APPENDIX

1. This and the ensuing discussion are drawn in part from D. M. Eddy, "Should We Change the Rules for Evaluating Medical Technologies?" in A. C. Gelijns, ed., *Medical Innovation at the Crossroads*, vol. 1. *Modern Methods of Clinical Investigation* (1990), 117–34.

2. E. O. Laumann, C. M. Masi, and W. W. Zuckerman, "Letters," *Journal of the American Medical Association* 278 (1997): 203.

3. For a full treatment, see M. Angell, *Science on Trial: The Clash of Medical Evidence and the Law in the Breast Implant Case* (1996).

4. M. Angell, "Overdosing on Health Risks," *New York Times Magazine*, 4 May 1997, 45.

INDEX